Surgical Revascularization of the Heart: The Internal Thoracic Arteries

Surgical Revascularization of the Heart: The Internal Thoracic Arteries

George E. Green, M.D.
Senior Attending Surgeon (Cardiothoracic Surgery)
St. Luke's/Roosevelt Hospital
And
Associate Clinical Professor of Surgery
Columbia University
New York, New York

Ram N. Singh, M.D.
Director, Cardiovascular Laboratory
St. Vincent Charity Hospital
Cleveland, Ohio
And former
Clinical Associate Professor of Medicine
University of Pittsburgh School of Medicine
And former
Director, Cardiac Catheterization Laboratory
Montefiore-University Hospital
Pittsburgh, Pennsylvania

J.A. Sosa, M.D.
Professor of Medicine and Radiology
Albany Medical College
And former
Director, Neil Hellman Cardiac Catheterization Laboratory
Albany Medical Center
Albany, New York

IGAKU-SHOIN • New York • Tokyo

Published and distributed by

IGAKU-SHOIN Medical Publishers, Inc.
One Madison Avenue, New York, N.Y. 10010

IGAKU-SHOIN Ltd.,
5-24-3 Hongo, Bunkyo-ku, Tokyo

Library of Congress Cataloging-in-Publication Data

Green, George E.
Surgical revascularization of the heart: the internal thoracic arteries / George E.
Green, Ram N. Singh, J. A. Sosa.
    p. cm.
    Includes index.
    1. Myocardial revascularization.   2. Internal thoracic artery—Surgery   I. Singh,
Ram N.,   II. Sosa, J. A.   III. Title.
    [DNLM: 1. Mammary Arteries—surgery.   2. Myocardial Revascularization.
    WG 169 G796s]
RD598.35.M95G74   1991
617.4′12059—dc20
DNLM/DLC
for Library of Congress

90-15655
CIP

ISBN: 0-89640-198-7 (New York)
ISBN: 4-260-14198-8 (Tokyo)

Printed and bound in the U.S.A.

10 9 8 7 6 5 4 3 2 1

Preface

In the fall of 1970 an editor from W.B. Saunders called. He suggested that we meet to discuss a book he proposed I write about the new field of coronary bypass surgery. We met at a quiet, elegant restaurant. I listened to the publishing possibilities and regretted that I didn't know enough to write a book about the new surgery.

In the summer of 1988 an editor from Igaku-Shoin called. The call was prompted by a *New York Times* article* concerning the surgical technique I had introduced in 1968. She proposed I write a book about it, and this time I was eager to proceed. The first requirement was a table of contents with an abstract of each chapter.

All coronary surgery has occurred during the twentieth century, most of it within the past 30 years. For example, in 1962 a friend and I traveled together to take our final examination by the American Board of Surgery. The examinations were oral. Each candidate was questioned by four panels of three examiners. On arrival we were separated. We didn't meet again until we left the building. He said, "One was outrageous, asking the wildest questions about the role of surgery in ischemic heart disease." We looked at each other in astonishment. Neither of us had ever thought of it.

Chapter 1 presents the history of the surgical effort in ischemic heart disease. Donald B. Effler was Chief of Cardiac Surgery at the Cleveland Clinic Foundation when I first heard him speak in 1965. He reported the Cleveland Clinic experience with Vineberg's operation to the 38th annual convention of the American Heart Association. He was lucid, forceful, and convincing. During the next decade, I often heard him speak and sometimes had the benefit of speaking with him. He was the evangelist of surgical revascularization. He sensed and preached its possibilities. He knew its requirements. His advice

---

*"Technique Changes in Bypass Surgery," by Lawrence K. Altman, M.D., *New York Times,* August 8, 1988, prompted the inquiry by Lila Maron of Igaku-Shoin. It also raised public consciousness and thereby hastened acceptance of a desirable change.

was sought throughout the world. I was delighted when he agreed to describe the development of surgical revascularization for this book.

In 1985 Frank Sims' view of the anatomical basis of atherosclerosis lit up my mental world. I had been working with the internal thoracic artery (ITA) for 20 years because it was resistant to atherosclerosis, but I had never known why. The joy of knowing came suddenly as I read Sims' work. Though sudden, that joy has been enduring.

I met Julio Sosa in 1969 at the 42nd annual convention of the American Heart Association, where I presented my early experience with ITA-coronary artery anastomoses. Sosa was interested in the procedure. He had been a medical student at McGill and had paid close attention to Vineberg's efforts to develop and validate myocardial implant techniques. Sosa was working with Mason Sones when Sones did the first angiographic studies of patients with Vineberg implants. Sosa wanted to do long-range angiographic evaluation of direct ITA anastomoses. His studies were in progress when Ram Singh began working in his laboratory at the Albany Medical Center. Singh too became fascinated by the ITA. He developed a special catheter for studying both the right and left ITAs from the right brachial approach. Singh left Albany to become director of a cardiac catheterization laboratory at the University of Pittsburgh. He instituted a series of basic studies on the angiographic anatomy of the ITA, and he continued collaborating with Sosa on postoperative evaluation. Together they collated the data that first documented the overwhelming superiority of ITA grafts.

I met Airlie Cameron in 1970 when I was appointed to St. Luke's Hospital to begin its coronary surgical program. She judged clinical follow-up crucial to evaluating surgical revascularization. Her clinical study began with the first operation at St. Luke's, on June 1, 1970, and included all patients operated on from then until December 31, 1972. She has evaluated these patients annually for 20 years, despite demanding commitments to the Coronary Artery Surgery Study and to clinical practice. By 1985 she had collated the data that statistically validated the long-term clinical advantages of ITA revascularizations over saphenous vein revascularizations. Moreover, she demonstrated that bilateral ITA revascularization was even more advantageous than single ITA revascularization. Because of her findings, I began using both ITAs in all patients in 1985.

George E. Green, M.D.
St. Luke's/Roosevelt Hospital
New York, New York

A Note on Nomenclature

In 1955 the International Anatomical Nomenclature Committee convened in Paris to unify anatomic nomenclature. The arteries about which so much is written in this book were designated internal thoracic arteries. Although surgeons and cardiologists commonly use the term internal mammary artery, we believe a better purpose will be served by using the terminology of the Nomina Anatomica of 1955 and its succeeding five editions.

Acknowledgment

Wild-Leitz USA, Inc. loaned the equipment for the micro photographs of this book. Dennis Corbisiero patiently instructed me in its use. Their generous help is gratefully acknowledged.

Contributors

Airlie A.C. Cameron, M.D.
Senior Attending Physician (Cardiology)
St. Lukes/Roosevelt Hospital
And
Associate Professor of Clinical Medicine
Columbia University
New York, New York

Donald Brian Effler, M.D.
Former Chairman, Department of Cardiothoracic Surgery
Cleveland Clinic Foundation
Cleveland, Ohio

Frank H. Sims, M.Sc., MB., Ch.B., Ph.D.
Honorary Research Fellow
Department of Pathology
University of Auckland School of Medicine
Auckland, New Zealand
And
Former Associate Professor of Pathology and Clinical Biochemistry
University of Toronto
Toronto, Ontario, Canada

Contents

CHAPTER ONE
HISTORICAL PHOTOGRAPHS

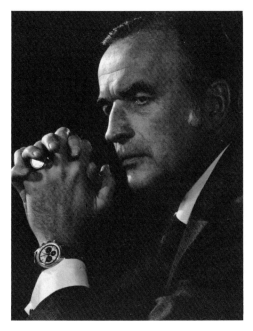

Donald B. Effler
1915–

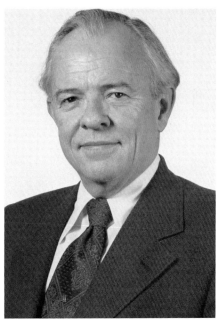

F. Mason Sones, Jr.
1919–1985

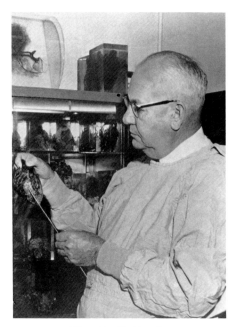

Claude S. Beck
1894–1971

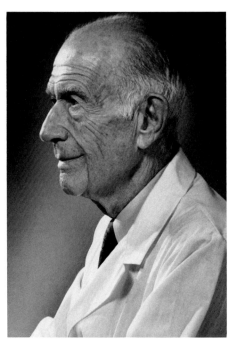

Arthur M. Vineberg
1903–1988

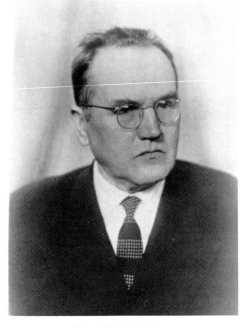

Vasilii I. Kolesov
1911–

Surgical Revascularization of the Heart: The Internal Thoracic Arteries

CHAPTER 1
History

DONALD BRIAN EFFLER

As Chief of Thoracic-Cardiovascular Surgery of the Cleveland Clinic Foundation, it was my frequent pleasure to welcome professional visitors from various parts of the world who were aware of our interest in revascularization surgery. These visits came with increasing frequency around 1960, a time at which we were increasingly identified with surgery for coronary artery disease, even though our surgical armamentarium in this field was restricted. Some of our visitors left lasting impressions; that is certainly true of Dr. George Green of New York City. In 1967 he was finishing his cardiothoracic surgical residency under Dr. Frank Spencer, but his research was being done in an experimental laboratory as he developed his approach to left internal thoracic artery–left anterior descending coronary artery anastomosis for direct myocardial revascularization. During his brief visit, Dr. Green showed me excellent movies of his operative approach and cineangiograms documenting the results. The Cleveland Clinic's facilities for the diagnosis and surgical treatment or coronary artery disease were expanding rapidly, and I was constantly on the lookout for young surgical talent. At the risk of offending Dr. Spencer, I suggested that Dr. Green think seriously about joining the Cleveland Clinic's team at the completion of his training program. We enjoyed a quiet dinner at my home in Shaker Heights, and the postprandial discussion lasted for several hours as I tried to convince this fine young man that there were particular advantages in major clinic practice that would help his career far more than he could expect in a busy city like New York. My recruitment efforts failed, but this did not impair a friendship that has persisted for well over 20 years. To me, it proved that I had good judgment as far as young surgical potential was concerned. By the time Green's textbook is published, I will have been retired for approximately 5 years and enjoying professional retirement at age 75. One cannot underestimate the influence of timing on a surgical career; this has certainly been true for me through luck and circumstance. During World War II, I ended my military career at Walter Reed General Hospital under the late Prof. Brian B. Blades, who was to remain my professional mentor until his

1

death at age 72 years. It was Dr. Blades who arranged my appointment to the Cleveland Clinic Foundation, where I would head the first Department of Thoracic Surgery. In 1945, cardiac surgery was limited to diseases of the pericardium and a few congenital heart problems that could be treated without extracorporeal circulation. Upon the advice of Dr. Blades, the Cleveland Clinic faculty agreed that I should spend a final year with Dr. John C. Jones, who was Chief of Thoracic Surgery at the Hospital of the Good Samaritan and, most important, Chief of Pediatric Congenital Heart Surgery at the Children's Hospital in Los Angeles. Dr. Jones became identified early with his work in patent ductus arteriosus and in coarctation of the aorta; his surgical experience closely paralleled that of Dr. Robert Gross in Boston. Initial exposure to Dr. Blades and then to Dr. Jones made me determined to head a department of thoracic-cardiovascular surgery at the Cleveland Clinic in 1949. Within 5 years, we had formed a basic team with Dr. Wilhelm Kolff and Dr. F. Mason Sones, Jr. Kolff established extracorporeal circulation in our laboratory and operating rooms, and Sones made monumental contributions in the development of selective coronary arteriography. In 1955 we introduced elective cardiac arrest as an adjunct to open-heart surgery for both congenital and acquired heart disease. Elective cardiac arrest, later to be called "cardioplegia," was an innovative approach to surgery that would make myocardial revascularization feasible from a technical standpoint. The subsequent development of Sones' technique for selective coronary arteriography in 1958 proved to be the catalyst for modern coronary artery surgery. I will be forever grateful to the Cleveland Clinic Foundation for providing a surgical atmosphere that instilled the desire for progress and development in fields that had not existed even a few months before our initial efforts. For this reason, I am taking the liberty of writing an introductory chapter in the first person and simply relating events that seem to be of critical importance at this time.

THE CORONARY PATIENT, CIRCA 1945

The diagnosis or the suspicion of coronary artery disease implied medical treatment. The diagnosis emphasized the presence of angina pectoris and was almost automatically established by evidence of a previous myocardial infarction and recovery. The most commonly used drug for symptomatic coronary patients was nitroglycerin or a related type of vasodilator. Basically, the medical therapy for the coronary patient was one that made the patient's life more bearable and possibly reduced the risk or delayed further infarction of the threatened myocardium. When the suspected patient was referred to the cardiologist, further emphasis was placed upon various risk factors that might effect the vulnerability to coronary disease and to a shorter life span. Control of correctable risk factors laid emphasis on reducing obesity, elimination of smoking, control of arterial blood pressure, and therapy for associated diseases that influenced the course of coronary atherosclerosis. Patients with diabetes mellitus and hypercholesterolemia were placed on an appropriate diet and medication in an effort to lower these risk factors. For patients who had endured and survived major infarctions, emphasis was placed upon a strict regimen to alter the lifestyle, reduce physical stress, and utilize digitalis when there was related cardiomegaly. The cardiologist relied heavily upon statistical patterns of coronary disease. These were used as guidelines to assess the patient's progress and, in a sense, to evaluate his or her long-term therapy. As would be expected, coronary patients frequently became dependent upon medical therapy, which could only modify to some degree the natural history of coronary disease. The mortality rates associated with medical therapy were well established by major insurance companies and were used to express the prognosis, particularly after a documented infarction.

In the years immediately following World War II, there was growing dissatisfaction with both the diagnosis and the medical management of coronary patients. A scattering of papers published in Europe and North America suggested that something might be accomplished by surgical intervention. This wishful thinking reflected the frustration and the limited success of overall medical therapy. Occasionally, references were made to papers written a decade or more before, suggesting that some form of sympathectomy, creation of vascular adhesions around the heart, or the use of omental grafts might stimulate inflammatory adhesions between the epicardium and pericardium. A review of the medical and surgical literature of that time gives no clue to the number of patients who actually sustained such operations, but they were attempted and the motives were well intended. Some of the procedures that were utilized and described were imaginative, to say the least. Multiple needle punctures of the left ventricular wall were tried in an effort to create new vascular channels between the left ventricular chamber and the ischemic myocardium. Epicardial abrasion was frequently used, supplemented with some form of poudrage or the application of phenol, which certainly would be classified as an irritant to the heart muscle. Several references are listed in the early literature, but these are probably far less in number and variety than the operations actually attempted. Looking back at the plight of the coronary patient, it does not come as a surporise that the search for a surgical solution to coronary artery disease is a story of frustration. Operations were used without any valid evidence that they could possibly accomplish their purpose. They were done simply because there was a need for surgical intervention of some kind. Whenever a rumor circulated that another inventive procedure for the treatment of coronary artery disease was being performed at some surgical center, surgeons became interested. The disturbing fact that the basic diagnosis of coronary artery disease was incapable of demonstrating the needs of the individual patient did not deter the quest for surgical treatment. If progress was to be made in the treatment of the coronary patient, something had to be done that would relieve myocardial ischemia by improving myocardial perfusion. Crucial to this effort was a means of direct assessment of diminished blood flow in viable myocardium. In addition, for treatment to be accomplished, there had to be a means of assessing the success or failure of the operative procedure. For this reason, it would seem pointless to present a collective review with innumerable references suggesting how much had been written and how little had been accomplished in revascularization surgery prior to 1945. Certainly, there is no need to emphasize the demand for such surgery and that the potential number of patients was incalculable. As far as surgical treatment was concerned, it is safe to say that some of the finest intellects in modern surgery were almost consumed with the quest for myocardial revascularization. For this reason, I have decided to abstract the surgical careers of three men whose work was outstanding at a time when surgery for coronary artery disease was generally unknown. Not one of the three ever achieved international recognition until late in life or after death.

CLAUDE SCHAEFFER BECK, CARDIAC SURGEON (1894–1971)

Dr. Claude Beck became a pioneer in the field of heart surgery before any type of formal training was available. At some point in midcareer, I enjoyed a private conversation with Dr. Beck, and he made the following statement: "After my initial surgical training, I was convinced that I would make my living in neurosurgery and never be identified with surgical treatment of certain heart diseases." He was influenced from the beginning by Dr. Elliot Cutler, who left Boston to become Professor of Surgery at Case Western Reserve University in Cleveland. This association prompted him to make various attempts at the surgical relief of mitral stenosis secondary to rheumatic heart disease. Beginning in 1930, Claude Beck made lasting contributions that will always identify him with heart surgery. The first definitive operation that bears his name was related to the surgical treatment of constrictive pericarditis. It was Beck and his co-workers who vividly described the triads of acute and chronic constrictive pericarditis. For the young medical student and surgical resident, these basic papers on Beck's observations and descriptions became required reading. It behooved the young candidate for examination by the American Board of Surgery and, later, the American Board of Thoracic Surgery to identify the triads for tamponade and chronic constrictive pericarditis. Not only did Beck describe the operative technique for each entity, but he clarified the clinical picture that enhanced recognition of the underlying pathology.

In a sense, Beck put the earliest form of heart surgery on a practical basis even though the diseased pericardium was only the periphery of the most important organ in the circulatory system. It was one thing to recommend an operative procedure that might provide an element of relief from pericardial constriction, but the fact that this surgeon could establish diagnostic triads to enhance recognition of the underlying problem is remarkable. In later years, it was my privilege to act as examiner for the American Board of Thoracic Surgery, and every new candidate was expected to understand the mechanisms of acute and chronic pericarditis even though he may never have seen a definitive operation for either entity. The fact that a single surgeon could make extraordinary contributions to the recognition and surgical treatment of acute or chronic pericarditis is in itself remarkable. Claude Beck did much more.

In 1903, Christen Thorel reported on a postmortem study in a patient who was found to have total occlusion of both the right and left main coronary arteries; there were dense adhesions around the heart, and it was assumed that the vascular adhesions had somehow provided collateral support to the coronary circulation. Beck reviewed this case study carefully with Professor Alan Moritz, a senior pathologist at Case Western Reserve University. If coronary atherosclerosis could obliterate the entire coronary artery supply and the patient could survive on the basis of vascular adhesions between the pericardium and epicardium, then this might offer a potential solution to progressive myocardial ischemia. This concept did not escape consideration by surgeons in England and other parts of the United States, and a number tried omental grafts to the viable myocardium in the hope that collateral blood supply could be encouraged. Many of these early operations were not documented because the results were less than impressive. Nevertheless, Beck persisted in experimental work with his typical tenacity, utilizing both omental grafts and abrasive techniques that would leave a raw surface on the myocardium and encourage (hopefully) vascular adhesions. The experimental surgery included free muscle grafts from the anterior chest wall, abrasion of the epicardial surface by rasps, and poudrage with powdered talc.

Beck's procedures were used clinically but sparingly. He continued experimenting and combined the intrapericardial abrasion procedures with partial occlusion of the coronary sinus. It had been suggested that partial occlusion of the coronary sinus would extract maximum amounts of the oxygen that remained in the returning venous blood. The clinical evaluation of surgical candidates at that time was less than exact, and the same can be said for those patients who were fortunate enough to survive this type of surgery. However, a number of patients seemed to improve after Beck's operation, and this encouraged continuation of the so-called Beck I procedure. Eleven of the patients Beck had operated on survived for 6 years, but none of these patients had the benefit of preoperative or postoperative coronary arteriography. Such studies were simply not available in 1954, yet Beck's enthusiasm was unflagging and he was determined to continue in this line of endeavor.

Beck raised funds to build an experimental laboratory complex that was a model for its time. Again, this was a reflection of his enthusiasm and determination to carry on work that had never been performed under similar circumstances. The basic facilities to perform high-grade animal surgery were the first order of business. Beck's associates included resident surgeons, qualified veterinary personnel, senior registered nurses, laboratory technicians, and postoperative recovery facilities that were not always available in hospitals that operated on human patients. Beck was convinced that the ideal animal for experimental coronary surgery was the purebred pit bull. These beautiful animals were treated with special care, and postoperative survival was a necessity if progress was to be made. In addition to the surgical facilities at Case Western Reserve University Hospital, Beck established a special farm where surviving dogs were boarded under the best available veterinary care. For the professional visitor, it was a privilege to observe Beck, his laboratory, his dedicated team of co-workers, and the beautiful animals that were reserved for surgical experimentation.

As might be expected, Dr. Beck was a man of fierce determination and did not take kindly to thoughtless, negative comments on his work. Although he could not provide definitive proof that revascularization of the ischemic myocardium was accomplished in any sense of the word, he did believe that he had to start somewhere, and if no one else would lead the way, he would do his best to accomplish this mission. Qualified visitors were treated with courtesy, and it was obvious that Beck wanted to provide proof of his conviction that something positive had already been attained. When I concluded my visit with Dr. Beck, he asked a firm question: "When are you going to start doing my operation?" He was referring to the Beck I procedure, and I did not think there was evidence to justify our involvement with his procedure at that point.

By 1948, Beck was determined to do some form of direct arterialization and decided that this would be accomplished by a graft between the descending aorta and the partially ligated coronary sinus. This operation would, in effect, create an arteriovenous fistula between these two structures. The procedure proved to be more difficult than had been anticipated because the arterial graft from the descending aorta to the transverse sinus involved unexpected technical problems. Initially, the Beck II operation was performed in separate stages, with insertion of the aortocoronary sinus graft at Stage I and then, at Stage II, partial ligation of the coronary sinus. Initially, the free graft entailed removal of the entire brachial artery, but this soon gave way to the use of a reversed saphenous vein graft. Although the procedure was simple in concept, the basic work involved was almost monumental, and considerable credit must be given to those who participated. As might be expected, the clinical results, in a relatively small series of cases, were disappointing. The Beck II procedure was shelved, and the less difficult Beck I procedure continued to have clinical application.

It should be mentioned that Beck's work in revascularization was sidetracked by his sudden interest in cardiopulmonary resuscitation. Postmortem examination of patients who had died unexpectedly in ventricular fibrillation frequently showed that the heart was basically sound and free of extensive coronary pathology. Under these circumstances, Beck described the situation as presenting "the heart that was too good to die." Although the problem was by no means resolved in its most sophisticated form by Beck's team, he did create a national awareness of the problem and the need for aggressive measures to provide cardiopulomonary resuscitation as we know it today.

Toward the end of his highly productive career, Claude Beck continued to observe his experimental animals and his postoperative patients, particularly those who had undergone the Beck I procedure for coronary insufficiency. Throughout the developmental and later years, he maintained his interest in surgery for acquired valvar disease that resulted in stenosis or combined stenosis and regurgitation at both the mitral and aortic levels. At about the time when his health was beginning to fail, I met him at a local meeting and congratulated him on his many contributions and his singular determination to improve the fate of the coronary artery patient. Claude Schaeffer Beck smiled at me and said quietly, "Not too bad for a man who originally made his living in neurosurgery, is it?" Throughout his long and productive career, Beck was an aggressive and imaginative surgeon. His primary goal, to develop a surgical treatment for coronary artery disease, was never achieved. But it is my contention this was not a failure by the man himself, but resulted from the simple fact that he was never given the benefit of selective coronary arteriography as it was to be developed by Sones and his Cleveland Clinic team. On many occasions, he overcame obstacles in his pursuit of surgical success but, unfortunately, the key ingredient of coronary arteriography was missing.

F. MASON SONES, JR., INVASIVE CARDIOLOGIST (1919–1985)

In 1950, Dr. Mason Sones had completed his basic training at Henry Ford Hospital in Detroit and was given the opportunity to start an invasive cardiology laboratory at the Cleveland Clinic Foundation. The original laboratory was small and equipped to study patients with congenital heart disease. The majority of patients referred for surgical consideration were those with atrial and ventricular septal defects, tetralogy of Fallot, and a gradually increasing number of patients who would be operated on later for patent ductus arteriosus and aortic coarctation. Due to the ingenuity of Dr. Wilhelm Kolff, extracorporeal circulation in its simplest form became available at the Cleveland Clinic around 1954; case selection was very limited as the young team of surgeons and cardiologists went through a form of basic training in this newly developing field. In 1955, the Cleveland Clinic team made a major breakthrough by introducing "Elective Cardiac Arrest" utilizing the Melrose concept of injecting potassium citrate into the aortic root to produce cardioplegia. Almost immediately, elective cardiac arrest improved the quality of the surgical product and attracted considerable attention at both national and international meetings of that time. The basic requirements for the ideal surgical field included (1) direct visualization, (2) absence of motion, and (3) minimal blood loss. These could be achieved only when the heart was put in a state of reversible cardiac arrest. It did not take long to develop the idea that the coronary arteries were accessible for surgical intervention, provided that an operation was available. At the same time, Sones and his colleagues were using the image intensifier that would augment fluoroscopy and record photographic images on 35mm cinefilm. The cardiovascular laboratory was located in the basement of the Cleveland Clinic and had almost unlimited capacity for expansion. Enlisting the help of major manufacturers of highly specialized equipment, the laboratory developed new image intensifiers until 1958, when the first Phillips 11-inch amplifier was installed. The equipment was large and so cumbersome that it was necessary to dig a pit beneath the table so that Sones could crouch and observe the field, much as a U-boat captain manned his periscope before an attack. It was necessary for the assistant injecting the contrast medium to follow verbal commands because he was unable to visualize any part of the radiographic screen. On October 24, 1958, a routine procedure was being done, with Sones in the pit and Dr. Royston Lewis as his assistant. Dr. Lewis recalls that he had prepared 40 cc of contrast medium for injection into the aortic root, a common practice that flooded the aortic root and permitted some visualization of both coronary arteries. This procedure was the state of the art for that time. Because of some transient distraction, Dr. Sones took his eye off the screen; at this precise moment, the catheter drifted into the ostium of the right coronary artery and descended for several centimers, a fact that was not appreciated immediately. When Dr. Lewis received his instructions to inject 40 cc of contrast medium into the aortic root, the entire dose was injected into the right coronary artery, well below the ostium and under very high pressure. It seemed obvious that this unintended dose injected into the right coronary artery would be unacceptable to the human heart, but subsequent events proved this assumption to be incorrect. The heart went into asystole for 6.5 seconds, but the patient did not lose consciousness and the heart returned to a sinus rhythm as the lights came on and Sones scrambled out of the pit. When quiet was restored and the film was reviewed, the first right selective coronary arteriogram had been performed and the value of the procedure (with a modified dosage of contrast medium) was recognized. A short time later, the 11-inch image intensifier was abandoned and the studies were performed with 5-inch equipment reproduced on 35mm film. As clinical experience increased, numerous lessons were learned concerning the anatomy and pathology of the coronary circulation; this, combined with left ventriculography, made up the routine study for a patient suspected of having coronary artery disease. Gone was the need for tedious dissection of the cadaveric heart and its coronary arterial circulation; the new technique of cinecoronary arteriography could be accomplished easily within 20 minutes. Equally important, the individual case could be studied and restudied until the needs of the patient were assessed clearly and rationally. By introducing selective coronary arteriography, Mason Sones and his colleagues created the modern era of revascularization surgery by providing accurate diagnosis and excellent appraisal of surgical treatment in the surviving patient. Almost from the beginning, it was my contention that left ventriculography described the state of health of the left ventricular myocardium and identified any impairment that might result from previous infarction or myocarditis in one form or another.

As the number of patients undergoing selective coronary arteriography at the Cleveland Clinic increased steadily, there were some cases where the problem was all too evident. This was true in major ostial lesions of both the dominant right and left coronary arteries. It was also true that patients with critical segmental stenosis of either coronary artery could be highly symptomatic and still have normal left ventricles, as demonstrated by ventriculography. Additional information revealed that an occasional patient, who insisted that he was totally asymptomatic, could have life-treatening major occlusions in what otherwise appeared to be normal coronary arterial circulation. The lessons to be learned from selective coronary arteriography in the hands of qualified people seemed to be almost endless. For the first time, the burden of action was placed squarely upon the cardiac surgeons, who had been provided with medical information beyond anyone's anticipation.

As more and more cases were carefully reviewed for possible surgical treatment, endarterectomy became a great temptation. Utilizing the map provided by arteriography, the segmental occlusion in a major coronary artery could be approached directly and curetted. But after a number of surgical attempts, pure endarterectomy was abandoned by the Cleveland Clinic group because of the so-called snowplow effect; that is, as the atheromatous obstruction was dissected free from the media, there could be a shearing effect upon the side branches and an undesired flap left at the distal end of the dissection. In small vessels, characteristic of the coronary arterial circulation, the snowplow effect could have a devastating impact upon the heart muscle supplied by the particular vessel. In 1962, the Cleveland Clinic team adopted a technique described earlier by Senning, in which the segmental obstruction was opened in a linear fashion to points above and below the block; this area was then enlarged in caliber by patch-graft reconstruction with vein or normal pericardium. More than 120 such operations were performed and enthusiasm mounted steadily, even though the number of patients with anatomy amenable to correction by this procedure were limited. All of us who were involved at that point were convinced that the possibility of myocardial revascularization was now established, and that it was simply a matter of improving and enlarging upon the number of techniques.

Dr. F. Mason Sones, Jr., had the invaluable ability to stimulate the productive work of other cardiologists, engineers, and imaginative people who could develop equipment and methods essential to his basic progress. As one of the involved surgeons, I consider this part of the chapter to be a direct tribute to Dr. Sones. Without him, the Cleveland Clinic participation would never have occurred.

ARTHUR M. VINEBERG, CARDIAC SURGEON (1903–1988)

Dr. Vineberg may well have been the first surgeon to accomplish myocardial revascularization by introducing arterial blood to an area of myocardial perfusion deficit. This is a broad statement, and I am sure it will be challenged by many who are as interested as and perhaps more knowledgeable than I regarding the history of coronary artery surgery. Those who might participate in this argument would contend that a wide variety of surgical procedures were introduced before Vineberg, and there is always the remote possibility that one or more of these might have accomplished its purpose; however, even if this were the case, there is no proof at this time. Unfortunately, in the days before coronary arteriography, most of the procedures advocated for myocardial revascularization were based upon unproven concepts. This was particularly true of abrasion of the epicardium, poudrage, acupuncture, omentopexy, bilateral internal thoracic artery ligation, and many other procedures in early surgical literature.

From the beginning, it had been appreciated that occlusive disease of epicardial arteries produced myocardial ischemia, particularly in the subepicardial distribution. Early on, it had been observed that intramyocardial branches of the coronary artery circulation were remarkably free of atherosclerotic obstruction. It had been recognized for centuries that angina pectoris was the classic symptom of coronary ischemia, and it was now generally agreed that this was produced by anaerobic metabolism in the affected heart muscle. If a surgical procedure was to help the patient with coronary artery disease, it would have to provide significant, perhaps measurable, improvement in myocardial perfusion, as shown by more than patient survival and relief of symptoms. It had long been noted that symptomatic patients lost their angina pectoris after surviving a myocardial infarction. The assumption was that recovery was due to the development of collaterals that made up for the preinfarction deficit. In the 1940s, it was common practice to congratulate the patient who had recovered from a myocardial infarction and was now asymptomatic. The assumption was that he was the fortunate one who had developed collaterals and was healthier than before the nearly disastrous infarction. Although the statistical evidence of the time suggested that this patient might sustain another perhaps fatal infarction within 2 or 3 years, it was conveniently disregarded in the interests of boosting morale. In the same way, when patients survived surgery intended to alleviate coronary arterial disease and became free of angina, the surgeon took credit for the positive result. It is no wonder that critical cardiologists found the surgeon's proof basically unacceptable.

Arthur M. Vineberg was born in Quebec in May 1903. According to his story, recounted to me a number of years ago, his grandfather escaped from Russia and emigrated to Montreal. He was adopted by a fur trapper in Quebec and changed his name from Orlofsky to Vineberg. He did well as a young trapper and later shipped furs to New York. The furs were made into hats, coats, and jackets and shipped to Europe for marketing. As a third-generation Vineberg, young Arthur proved to be an apt medical student and a determined surgical resident. In 1945, Vineberg presented his thesis of revascularization with the internal thoracic artery implant. This concept was crystal clear to him but not to most of his peers. As a young thoracic surgeon immediately after World War II, it was my privilege to attend a number of annual meetings of the American Association for Thoracic Surgery and the American College of Surgeons. Occasionally Vineberg appeared on one of these programs and presented his work on internal thoracic artery implantation as a means of myocardial revascularization. I found his work of interest, but it was obvious that most of his peers gave little thought to it or to any other form of so-called revascularization surgery. Surgeons who were leaders in their field had ample opportunity to listen to Vineberg and to read his papers, but few inquired into the factors that influenced a favorable response to an internal thoracic implant. This is understandable because the scenario was like something out of science fiction, and until there was visual evidence or a means of measuring flow in a working implant, there was little reason to accept Vineberg's hypothesis. Survival of a small number of patients was certainly not enough.

Perhaps if our leading chest surgeons and cardiologists after World War II had devoted a bit more time and interest to Vineberg's presentations, others would have considered the subject in more detail. First of all, the internal thoracic artery, as Vineberg pointed out, is unique in many respects; some observers referred to it as a "primitive artery." Arteriosclerosis in this pair of intrathoracic arteries, even in older patients with diffuse disease elsewhere, is most unusual. Vineberg pointed out that it had unique properties: The small intercostal side branches were capable of proliferation after implantation, and the main internal thoracic artery increased in caliber when successfully implanted in the myocardial tunnel.

Vineberg made these observations in the experimental laboratory by injecting the vessel with Schlessinger mass. These unique properties of the internal thoracic artery after successful implantation were to be demonstrated repeatedly by postoperative arteriograms that showed a patent implant with internal thoracic-coronary anastomoses. Vineberg relied heavily on the observation that viable myocardium contains sinusoids consisting of endothelium-lined spaces in the muscle of the left ventricular myocardium. He believed that these sinusoids accounted for the fact that intramyocardial hematoma is rarely encountered after surgical trauma to the left ventricle. He reasoned that the artery with bleeding side branches could be implanted in viable myocardium and that the procedure would be tolerated well under general anesthesia. If the artery had a normal blood pressure and there was lower pressure in the arteries at the site of implantation, then functional demand would stimulate the side branches to proliferate and communicate directly with the comparable side branches of coronary arteries. Many qualified surgeons found this reasoning difficult to accept. The fact that experimental animals survived the operation seemed little justification for clinical application. However, a few Canadian and American surgeons were impressed with Vineberg's work, and some of them did perform operations on patients in both countries.

Vineberg was a tenacious man. He never questioned his experimental observations and was determined to establish some acceptable form of proof. Since coronary arteriography as we know it today, did not exist, it was necessary for him to track down patients who had survived his operation and had died suddenly of unrelated causes. When he was able to salvage a postmortem heart soon after death, he injected the internal mammary artery with contrast medium (Schlessinger mass) to form a cast of the arterial implant. Obviously, this was cumbersome and difficult, but it attested to his energy and determination. To his own satisfaction, he did have specimens that radiographically demonstrated the connection between the implant and the coronary artery.

Vineberg later developed a technique for applying ameroids to specific branches of the left coronary artery in dogs. The ameroid was a metal ring that encased a porous material that was hydroscopic. A linear slit in the metal ring allowed the ameroid to be slipped around the dissected portion of the coronary artery. As the hydroscopic material expanded by absorbing body fluid, the arterial lumen became progressively constricted until a gradient was created and ischemia resulted. In this way, Vineberg successfully created localized coronary insufficiency and a predictable myocardial perfusion deficit. An artery implant was then placed in an area of anticipated myocardial perfusion deficit. This experimental surgery took on a glamour that had a distinctly negative impact on many casual observers. It seemed that the harder Vineberg worked to pursue his goal, the more difficult it became to convince the skeptics.

Around 1960, I had the privilege of visiting Vineberg at McGill University and saw the Vineberg technique demonstrated in his laboratory. To this day, I am impressed with the skill and determination of this experimental heart surgeon. The dogs who had had ameroids applied earlier were carefully separated, and they would become predictably symptomatic and susceptible to sudden death if involved in a simple dog fight. The dogs who had received an ameroid and then an internal mammary implant were the treasures of his collection; they were capable of surviving the myocardial ischemia produced by ameroids.

Upon returning to Cleveland, I gave a detailed report to our team of surgeons and cardiologists. My enthusiasm for what I had seen in Vineberg's laboratory prompted considerable interest, but it was agreed that the Cleveland Clinic team would defer clinical application until it was possible to document the success of the Vineberg procedure in the human patient. We did not wait long. In 1962, three patients were referred from Canada; they had been operated upon by Dr. Wilfred Bigelow in Toronto General Hospital. These were followed by several patients referred by Vineberg himself. The patients were selected because they were survivors of internal thoracic artery implant procedures and were free of their preoperative symptoms. It is safe to say that these patients were the first to undergo internal thoracic arteriography and coronary arteriography to evaluate Vineberg's procedure. The first three patients were found to have patent internal thoracic artery implants and visible collateral communications between the implanted artery and the anterior descending branch of the left coronary artery. This was proof positive that Vineberg's hypothesis was valid and that true myocardial revascularization had been accomplished in human patients. Looking back, it was an ironic victory because the extensive and frustrating work of Vineberg and his colleagues had gained so little acceptance by surgeons in the United States and Canada. But in a short time, dramatic proof was made available by combined internal thoracic-coronary arteriography utilizing Sones' technique.

The dramatic development following Sones' study of the Canadian patients had an electrifying effect upon the Cleveland Clinic team. The clear knowledge that Vineberg's hypothesis was valid and that his operation could solve problems in many coronary patients galvanized the surgeons and cardiologists of the Cleveland Clinic. In 1962, we started an escalating series of operations utilizing the left internal thoracic artery combined with epicardial abrasion and free omental graft. As the number of cases grew, there came to be increasing doubt about the value of abrasion and the omental graft as an adjunct to revascularization. Finally, surgeons became totally dependent upon internal thoracic artery implantation itself.

Initially, the left internal thoracic artery was taken down from the chest wall in the manner described by Vineberg. The vessel was denuded, and the side branches were carefully protected until the distal artery could be divided and then the side branches snipped to permit free bleeding. When the artery was carefully removed from the anterior chest wall, at least two or three of the paired bleeding side branches were salvaged. The distal end of the artery with bleeding side branches was then implanted in the myocardial tunnel, and the presence of "bleeders" encouraged anticipation of early communication with branches of the obstructed coronary artery. At this time, it was obvious that true revascularization would not be a reality until enough time elapsed for intramyocardial communication to develop. It was recognized that the immediate postoperative period would be the most logical time for perioperative infarction to occur. For this reason, emphasis was placed upon protection by general anesthesia and prolonged sedation during the recovery period. Originally, it was thought that interarteriolar communications would require months to develop, but with increasing experience, it became apparent that the time factor varied considerably with the individual. As more patients underwent postoperative arteriography and internal thoracic arteriography, it became apparent that such interarteriolar communications might develop within a few weeks rather than months. It also became apparent that the implant itself could be modified to reduce the danger of injuring the all-important side branches prior to implantation. Based on the observations of Sewell, the internal thoracic artery was taken down as a pedicle, with no effort made to expose the naked internal thoracic artery itself. This pedicle required a larger intramyocardial tunnel, but retraction of the internal thoracic artery was less likely to occur, and on postoperative evaluation it seemed that the quality of the implant finally obtained was better than that achieved with the naked artery technique.

Eventually, most members of the Cleveland Clinic team utilized a compromise procedure in which the internal thoracic bundle was taken down on a fat pedicle and then tailored to meet the requirements of the intramyocardial tunnel created by dissection. The so-called Vineberg-Sewell pedicle became standard, and postoperative results were generally improved. Although the internal thoracic artery pedicle was mobilized from the level of the first rib to its full length, there was little tendency for the artery to retract, and the intramyocardial tunnels could be made longer to accommodate more side branches. Also, it became apparent that almost the entire left ventricular myocardium was accessible for implantation. In cases of triple-vessel coronary disease, both the right and left internal thoracic arteries could be utilized during the same procedure or even in a two-stage procedure in which one bundle was implanted on the anteroapical portion of the left ventricle while the other, usually the left, was placed on the posterolateral aspect of the left ventricle. The Vineberg approach to revascularization with the internal thoracic artery implant, or implants, requires a certain amount of surgical dexterity and the best supportive anesthesia. Resident surgeons were first taught to harvest the internal thoracic artery pedicles, which were then wrapped in gauze soaked with papaverine. Creation of the intramyocardial tunnels required skill that came with experience and repetition.

Between 1962 and 1968, over 2,000 patients underwent internal thoracic artery implant procedures in the Cleveland Clinic Hospital. Survivors of these procedures were encouraged to return for arteriography and appraisal of the result obtained. In the first 300 patients evaluated for single implant procedures, the graft patency rate exceeded 90%; a breakdown of the patent implant record showed that over 50% of these patients had demonstrable side branches that communicated with the obstructed coronary artery. These patients had received true myocardial revascularization. A significant segment of patent implants merely had the so-called myocardial blush. In these implants the myocardium was receiving appreciable contrast medium, but the exact arteriolar communications were difficult to visualize.

The success rate of internal thoracic artery implant procedures after 5 years of clinical application in the Cleveland Clinic proved beyond question that Vineberg's original hypothesis of revascularization was sound and that many patients received benefit from this operative approach. Perhaps the most striking results were those obtained in patients in whom basic coronary artery disease progressed to total occlusion of the left and/or right main coronary ostia; yet these patients survived because the internal thoracic arteries had supplied gradually increasing volumes of arterial blood to distal segments of the occluded coronary arteries. In addition, the luminal size of the internal thoracic artery in these vital implants had significantly increased as the demand for blood kept pace with ostial occlusion. Needless to say, these superb clinical results were not always predictable when the patients were initially evaluated and selected for surgical treatment by the implant technique, but the large Cleveland Clinic experience involving numerous surgeons established the Vineberg hypothesis beyond all question.

At this writing, there are patients who have survived with patent internal thoracic artery implants for 25 years; some of them are now in their eighth and ninth decade of life. We have learned that the life span of the average saphenous vein bypass graft cannot be compared with that of successful internal mammary implant. A successful bypass graft usually yields its highest flow and most effective revascularization immediately after the procedure. Since the internal thoracic implant has the capacity for accommodating to greater demands for arterial blood supply in the affected myocardium, the volume of flow through the implant can increase over time. This is seen when patients undergo repeated studies, and it has been demonstrated that the internal thoracic artery itself increases in caliber as the demands made upon the graft become greater. Cardiologists in Sones' laboratory demonstrated time and again that patients survived total occlusion of both the right and left coronary ostia because successful bilateral implants carried increasing coronary flow through anastomotic channels created by implantation. Great credit must be given to Dr. Arthur Vineberg for his initial hypothesis and for his determination to prove that true revascularization could be accomplished through a seemingly indirect surgical approach.

PROFESSOR VASILII E. KOLESOV, CARDIAC SURGEON (1904–)

This introductory chapter has been written about three professional men who were personal acquaintances and friends of mine: Dr. Claude Schaeffer Beck, Dr. F. Mason Sones, and Dr. Arthur M. Vineberg. Unfortunately, I have never had the opportunity to meet Professor Vasilii Kolesov of Leningrad. His professional work and interests first came to my attention in 1967, when I received a personal letter plus Kolesov's manuscript from Brian Blades, editor of the *Journal of Thoracic and Cardiovascular Surgery*. Recently, I have received much information from Dr. Kolesov's biographer, Dr. Andrew S. Olearchyk, who now lives in Philadelphia. Original papers by Kolesov and subsequent private communication from Olearchyk provide the basis for the final portion of this chapter.

The 1967 paper by Kolesov was entitled "Mammary Artery–Coronary Artery Anastomosis as a Method of Treatment for Angina Pectoris." It described Kolesov's concepts of direct revascularization surgery and his limited clinical experience with the left internal thoracic artery–coronary artery anastomosis. Again, it is important to mention that coronary arteriography (Sones' technique) was not available to Professor Kolesov, and the case selection had to be based upon the electrocardiogram (ECG) conventional cardiologic evaluation, and even direct inspection of the heart during operation. Evaluation of the surgical procedure depended on patient survival and on ECG and symptomatic changes. After reading this paper, it seemed to me that Kolesov, like Beck and Vineberg, was ahead of his time, and that he would have difficulty proving to a critical observer that (1) the operation was truly indicated and (2) the benefits attributed to the operation resulted from patent grafts and direct revascularization. It is interesting that a Russian surgeon working in Leningrad and performing operative procedures destined for the future was already publishing his work and his appraisal of the basic concept. It is safe to say that readers of Kolesov's 1967 paper may have had a tendency to downplay his surgical efforts and those of the Leningrad team. Certainly, the same can be said of most of the American and Canadian surgeons who earlier passed judgment on Beck and Vineberg.

In 1988, the *Journal of Cardiovascular Surgery* published a second article describing the pioneer work of Kolesov and dealing with his initial efforts to develop direct revascularization by an internal thoracic artery graft to a major branch of the coronary artery system. This article was submitted by Dr. Olearchyk, and I have relied strongly upon him as my primary source of information. It is obvious that Olearchyk developed an early and intense interest in coronary revascularization surgery and kept abreast of significant developments and published papers from both Europe and North America. He had been exposed to Kolesov and was aware of his techniques beginning in February 1964. It is obvious that he developed a high regard for Kolesov and is convinced that much of his early work was original and deserving of special commendation in world literature on revascularization surgery. On the basis of my own limited observations and general knowledge, I am inclined to agree.

Vasilii I. Kolesov was born on September 24, 1904, in the Vologda Province of Russia. He graduated from the Second Leningrad Medical Institute in 1931. After going through basic training in a number of institutions, he served as a senior surgeon at an evacuation hospital during the siege of Leningrad (1941–1944). According to Olearchyk, his major medical responsibilities included the position of Surgeon and Chief (1941–1951) of the Central Military Group and then of Chairman of Military Surgery at the Medical Institute in Kharkiv, the Ukraine. In 1953, he was appointed Chairman of the Department of Surgery at the First Leningrad Medical Institute of I.P. Pavlov. He is said to have written over 300 publications, including 13 monographs, among these "The Surgery of Coronary Arteries of the Heart" in 1977. At this writing, Dr. Kolesov is retired but still lives in Leningrad and retains an active interest in the development of revascularization surgery.

It is difficult for me to analyze Kolesov's clinical experience with coronary artery surgery, as his technical approaches were somewhat different from those used in the United States. The early operations utilized a left anterior thoracotomy and were performed without extracorporeal circulation. The selection of the surgical candidate is not clear, but strong emphasis was placed upon symptoms and extensive ECG findings. As stated before, selective coronary arteriography was not available to Kolesov, and the initial operative procedures were performed with the beating heart under ordinary anesthesia. Like many other Russian surgeons, Kolesov was interested in mechanical suturing techniques and used a number of specially constructed instruments that were devised by engineers and produced in Leningrad. His early writings discuss in detail the technical aspects of these devices. It would seem likely that some of his earlier operations were observed by visiting American or Canadian surgeons, but this is not entirely clear. With increasing experience, Kolesov seemed to favor operative procedures that utilized both mechanical suturing and direct vessel suturing. Apparently, the majority of operations involved the left internal thoracic artery and a major branch of the left anterior descending coronary artery with the beating heart. According to his descriptions, as translated by Olearchyk, a number of the basic procedures were performed on patients with unstable angina, and at least one or two were recovering from myocardial infarction.

By September 26, 1969, Kolesov had reported on 45 patients who had undergone single and bilateral internal thoracic-coronary artery grafts, with a mortality rate of 14.9%. Strengthened by this initial experience, Kolesov extended the operative procedures over the next 7 years and operated on 132 patients. As stated in his earlier papers, Kolesov emphasized that the majority of his patients were not only symptomatic but had had one or more myocardial infarctions prior to surgery. In discussing this second series of 132 patients, I find it of particular interest that he states, "Preoperative evaluation consisted of symptomatology, ECG with multiple leads, stress testing, and cardiac catheterization with coronary arteriography." It is not clear from the information provided, and it would be very interesting to know, when coronary arteriography became available to Kolesov and to what extent it was used for evaluation and postoperative study of surviving patients.

Those of us who were performing heart surgery from 1960 to 1967 are well aware that surgical practices varied tremendously throughout the world. Olearchyk makes the rather strong statement that Kolesov's Department of Surgery was the only center in the world where coronary revascularization was systematically performed between 1964 and 1967. Actually, this statement is easily challenged, because a variety of revascularization procedures, including coronary endarterectomy, coronary arteriotomy with patch-graft reconstruction, angioplasty under direct vision, and interposed vein grafts, were being used in the United States and Canada. I am certain of this because of personal involvement at the Cleveland Clinic. It should also be mentioned that Vineberg's implant procedures were being done in increasingly large numbers. I am willing to concede that Vasilii Kolesov may have done the first successful internal thoracic-coronary artery anastomosis, but unfortunately the angiographic capability that could have supported this claim was not available to him.

It is not the purpose of this chapter to lay a claim for any individual who might have introduced a successful revascularization procedure. It has been written in response to the request for my description of how surgery for coronary revascularization developed. And it is my intention to recognize Dr. George E. Green of New York City, as one who has made a major contribution in the development of internal thoracic-coronary artery surgery. I know this to be true, because I remember well reviewing those beautiful cineangiographic studies he made in 1967.

CHAPTER **2**

The Pathology of the Internal Thoracic Artery and Its Contribution to the Study of Atherosclerosis

FRANK H. SIMS

THE INTERNAL THORACIC ARTERY (ITA)

Histological Features

Despite its comparatively small size, this artery is closely related in structure to the great vessels such as the aorta, the brachial artery, and the common carotid artery—the so-called elastic arteries. Figure 2–1 shows the internal thoracic artery (ITA) of an infant aged 4 months, and Fig. 2–2 shows a more detailed appearance of the wall of this vessel from a child 4 years of age.

In conventional terminology, the arterial wall is composed of three compartments, named from the lumen outward: the intima, bounded externally by the internal elastic lamina (IEL); the media, limited externally by the external elastic lamina (EEL); and the adventitia.

The Intima

The lumen of the ITA is lined by a single layer of regularly arranged, flattened endothelial cells elongated in the direction of blood flow (Figs. 2–3 and 2–4). These cells are close to the IEL and separated from it by a space which is narrow in the young subject and contains collagen fibers and proteoglycan matrix. The IEL is a thick lamina of elastin which appears almost continuous by light microscopic examination and separates the intimal compartment from the media (Fig. 2–2).

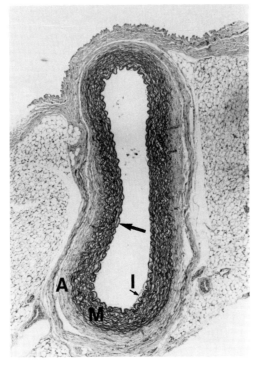

FIGURE 2-1 Section of the ITA of a male infant aged 4 months. Small arrow = intima; M = media; A = adventitia; large arrow = IEL. Orcein-Haematoxylin (Hx), 50×.

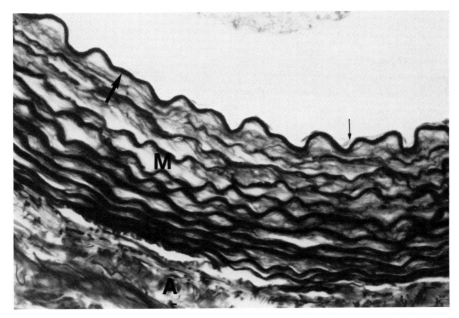

FIGURE 2-2 The ITA of a male child aged 4 years. Small arrow = intima; M = media; A = adventitia; large arrow = IEL. Orcein-Hx, 350×.

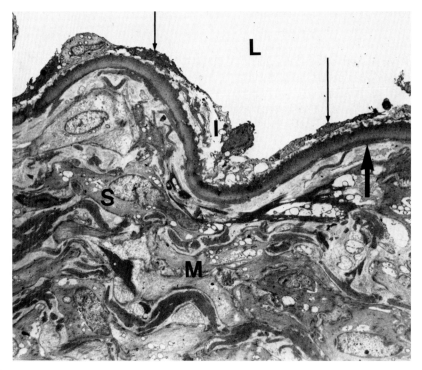

FIGURE 2-3 The ITA of a male child aged 2 years. Transmission electron micrograph (TEM). L = lumen; I = intima; M = media; small arrows = endothelial cells; S = SMC of media; large arrow = IEL. Orcein, uranyl acetate, lead citrate, 1,900×.

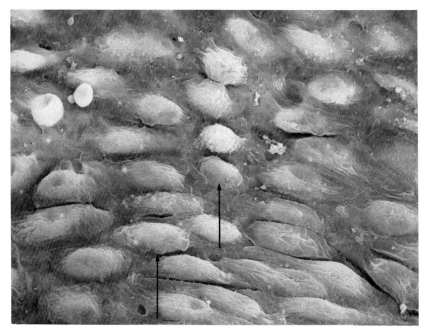

FIGURE 2-4 The endothelial surface of the ITA of the subject in Fig. 2-3 viewed by scanning electron microscopy (SEM). The nuclei of the endothelial cells (arrows) are prominent due to the stronger emission of back-scattered electrons. 355×.

The Media

This is composed of many layers of elastin (about nine in the first years of life) (Fig. 2–2) separated from each other by smooth muscle cells (SMC), collagen fibers, and proteoglycan matrix (Fig. 2–3). In contrast to the IEL, these elastin layers are discontinuous and are linked together by fine elastin interconnecting fibers. The SMC are close to these interconnecting elastin fibers, and both are arranged circumferentially when the arterial wall is under physiological pressure. Collagen fibers are present in the spaces between the lamellae of elastin and the SMC, and are circumferentially arranged when the wall is distended. The media is a two-phase structure whose strength in resisting the pulsatile pressure of the blood is due to the combination of the network of elastin lamellae and interconnecting fibers, coupled with the circularly arranged collagen fibers. The elastic appears to distribute the stress and contribute to the strength of the wall, the collagen providing the component with the highest tensile strength. It has been shown that this type of arterial wall expands readily with lower pressures, but in the physiological range and above, it is very resistant to further dilatation.[1-4]

Adventitia

The adventitia is similar in structure in all the larger arteries (Fig. 2–2). It is composed of discontinuous elastin fibers, the EEL, scattered throughout a strong collagenous envelope merging without demarcation into the surrounding perivascular connective tissue. The collagenous fibers run obliquely and have a longitudinal strengthening effect which resists lengthening of the arterial wall.[4]

Comparison With Other Vessels

Although the ITA closely resembles other elastic arteries in structure, its IEL appears to be more robust and more completely formed than that of most of the other vessels. Figure 2–5 shows the aortic wall of a 1-month-old infant, and Figure 2–6 shows the common carotid artery of an infant aged 6 months. The IELs of these vessels show noticeable discontinuities, although, as with the ITA, the media is composed of many lamellae of elastin separated by SMC and collagen.

The structure of the elastic arteries contrasts sharply to that of the medium-sized or muscular arteries, the media of which is composed almost entirely of SMC separated by collagen fibers and proteoglycan matrix. Only a small and variable amount of fragmented, attenuated elastin is present in the media of these vessels (Figs. 2–7 and 2–8). The intima of the muscular arteries also is little more than a potential compartment in the young subject, the endothelium lying in close approximation to the IEL. The adventitia is the same strong collagenous sheath containing variable amounts of elastin which is seen in all the larger arteries.

In these vessels, the IEL also shows great variability, frequently containing obvious discontinuities, particularly in the coronary artery. Figures 2–9 and 2–10 show such discontinuities in the coronary and splenic arteries. Cerebral

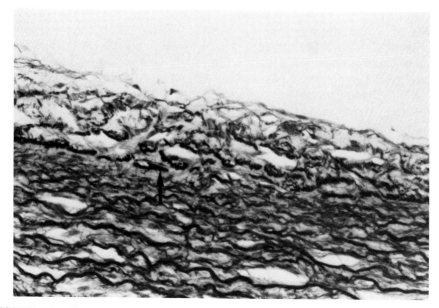

FIGURE 2-5 Aortic wall of an infant aged 1 month. There are obvious defects in the IEL (arrow) and well-developed intimal thickening. Orcein-Hx, 350×.

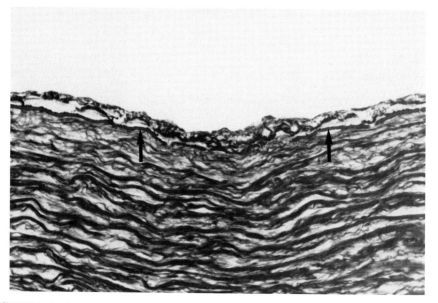

FIGURE 2-6 Common carotid artery of an infant aged 5 months. Arrows show the IEL, which is defective. Early intimal thickening is present. Orcein-Hx, 350×.

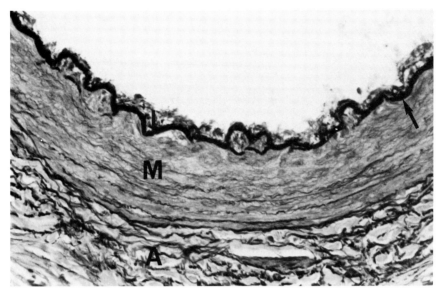

FIGURE 2–7 Coronary artery of a female infant aged 2 months. I = intima; M = media; A = adventitia; arrow = IEL showing obvious discontinuities. Orcein-Hx, 350×.

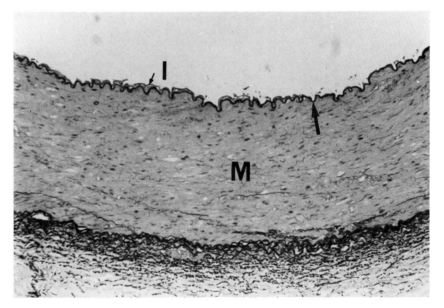

FIGURE 2–8 Splenic artery of a male aged 23 years. I = intima; M = media. In the area shown, there is incipient intimal thickening (arrow). Orcein-Hx, 80×.

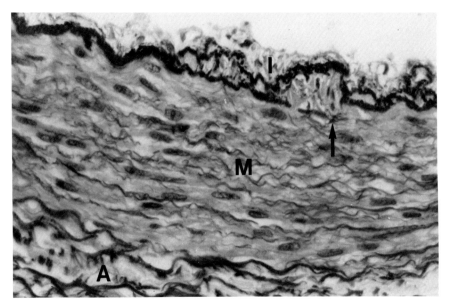

FIGURE 2-9 Higher-power view of Fig. 2-7 showing discontinuities of the IEL (arrow). The plane of the section passes through only one of the two gaps in the IEL. I = intima; M = media; A = adventitia. Orcein-Hx, 500×.

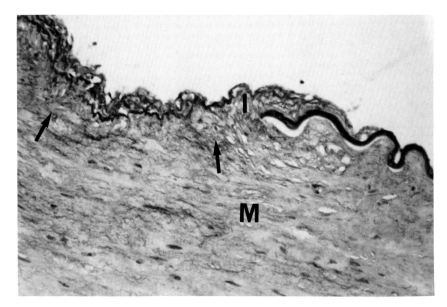

FIGURE 2-10 Higher-power view of Fig. 2-8 showing similar discontinuities of the IEL. I = intima; M = media; arrows = discontinuity of the IEL. Orcein-Hx, 500×.

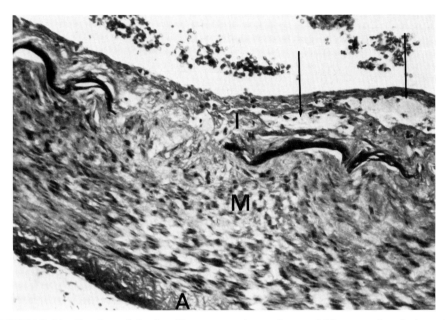

FIGURE 2–11   Section of the basilar artery of a male aged 35 years. I = intima; M = media; A = adventitia. Note the foamy macrophages in the thickened intima (arrows). The IEL presents a gap through which medial cells are growing, Verhoeff's elastin-Hx, 200×.

arteries such as the basilar, anterior, and posterior cerebral arteries have a very thick IEL, which, however, presents isolated defects (Fig. 2–11). The visceral arteries in general have better-formed IELs but still show defects even in younger age groups.

The larger veins resemble the muscular arteries in many respects but also show significant differences. The luminal surface of the intima is covered by a single layer of regularly arranged endothelium separated only slightly from the IEL in the young subject by loose matrix containing collagen. The IEL is poorly formed, with extensive discontinuities (Fig. 2–12). The media is formed largely of collagen, with small, variable numbers of SMC and fine, discontinuous lamellae of elastin. The adventitia is also formed of collagen and discontinuous lamellae of elastin. The media of veins from the lower extremity, such as the saphenous vein, have more smooth muscle than those from the upper part of the body. Valves are present in the veins from the dependent portion of the body and oppose reflux of blood toward the periphery. They are composed of a fine elastin lamella on the distal aspect, covered by a collagenous matrix proximally, with the free surface covered by endothelial cells (Fig. 2–13).

Changes in the Structure of the ITA Throughout Life

Although the ITA is almost perfectly formed at birth, and although this vessel does not develop significant thickening of the intima in younger age groups,

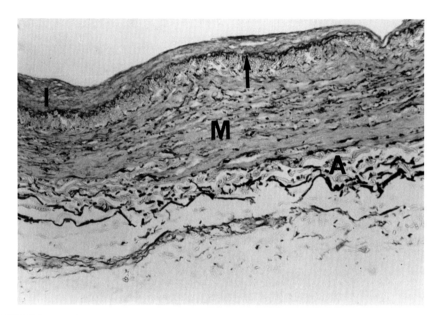

FIGURE 2–12 Saphenous vein of a male aged 52 years. I = intima; M = media; A = adventitia; arrow = IEL, which is poorly formed, with numerous gaps. The media is composed of collagen and SMC. Orcein-Hx, 80×.

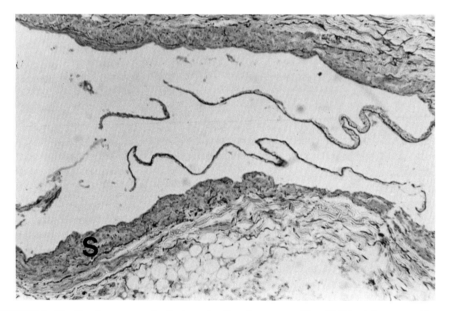

FIGURE 2–13 Saphenous vein in longitudinal section. The SMC of the wall (S) are shown here in cross-section. The leaflets of a valve are present in the section. Orcein-Hx, 80×.

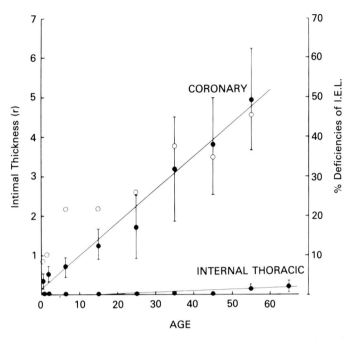

FIGURE 2–14 Graph showing the variation with age of the intimal thickness of the anterior descending coronary artery and the ITA from Ref. 6. Intimal thickness (r) is determined as follows:

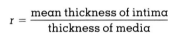

$$r = \frac{\text{mean thickness of intima}}{\text{thickness of media}}$$

such changes do eventually occur in some older subjects. This contrasts with other arteries of medium and large size, which develop intimal thickening at an early age that progresses throughout life. Figure 2–14 illustrates graphically the rate of intimal thickening of the ITA compared with that of the anterior descending coronary artery.

Intimal thickening of the ITA, like that of other arteries, is due to the growth of SMC from the media through gaps in the IEL into the intimal compartment[5,6] (Figs. 2–9 to 2–11). With the ITA, such defects occur more frequently in older age groups, due probably to the degeneration of elastin which is known to occur with advancing age.[7] These changes tend to occur particularly near the origin of the vessel from the subclavian artery (Figs. 2–15 and 2–16). In advanced cases, the histological picture of the intima is similar to that of typical atherosclerosis in other susceptible vessels, with lipid deposition and areas of necrosis (Fig. 2–17). Some individuals, however, retain a well-formed IEL and show minimal intimal thickening even at an advanced age (Fig. 2–18). Other older subjects may have very little elastin in the media of the ITA, perhaps due to degeneration of the medial lamellae. In such cases, if the IEL is well formed, there may be no significant intimal thickening (Fig. 2–19).

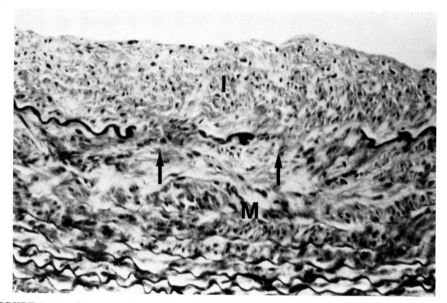

FIGURE 2–15 Cross-section of the wall of the ITA of a female aged 58 years. The section shows defects of the IEL (arrows) through which medial cells are entering the thickened intima (I). M = media. Verhoeff's elastin-Hx, 240×.

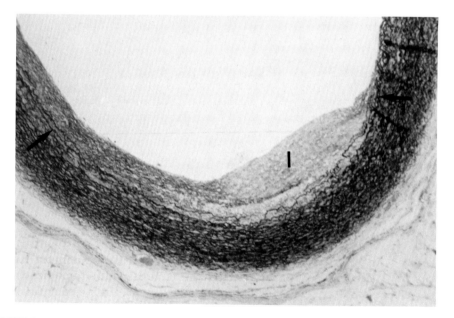

FIGURE 2–16 Intimal thickening in the ITA of a male aged 58 years. There is obvious disorganization of the IEL (arrows) and intimal thickening (I). Media and adventitia are normal. Orcein-Hx, 50×.

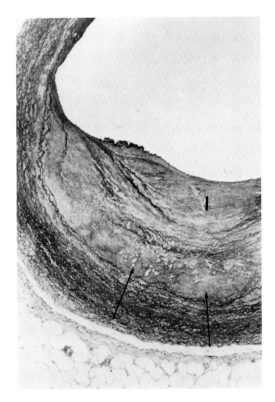

FIGURE 2–17 Greater intimal thickening of the ITA, also from a male aged 58 years. A typical atheromatous plaque is present, with an area of degeneration and lipid deposition (arrows) with overlying fibroelastic tissue (I). The IEL is disorganized. Orcein-Hx, 50×.

It thus appeasrs that the ITA behaves the same way as any other artery when there are discontinuities in the IEL. Therefore, if there are no defects in the IEL, there is no intimal thickening.

Development of the ITA

It is interesting to speculate on the reasons for the relative freedom of the ITA from arterial disease in comparison with other arteries of the same size in the same subject, since all systemic arteries are perfused with the same blood at essentially the same pressure. The evidence which is emerging, and which is discussed in more detail in the following sections, strongly suggests that the formation of a better IEL is the key factor in the resistance of this vessel to the development of arterial disease.

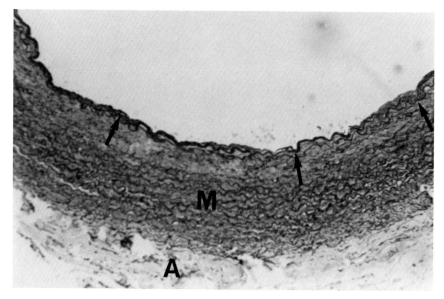

FIGURE 2-18 The ITA of a female aged 96 years showing minimal intimal thickening. The IEL is well preserved (arrows), the media and adventitia are essentially normal. Orcein-Hx, 80×.

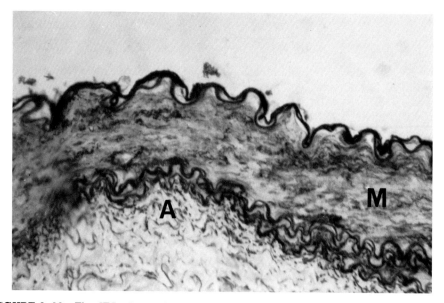

FIGURE 2-19 The ITA of a male aged 60 years. There is degeneration of many of the medial lamellae of elastin, leaving a media composed predominantly of SMC (M). The IEL is well preserved, and there is no significant intimal thickening. A = adventitia. Orcein-Hx, 200×.

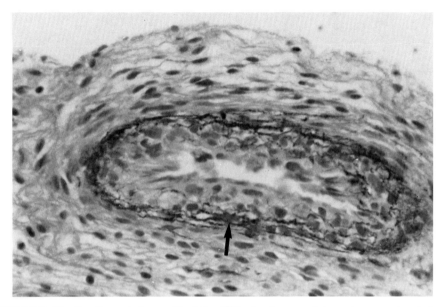

FIGURE 2-20 Section of the wall of the ITA of a human fetus at approximately 11 weeks gestation. Note the absence of an IEL but considerable elastin deposition in the surrounding EEL (arrow). Orcein-Hx, 500×.

The question then arises, why during development is the IEL of this vessel better formed than that of others?

Studies of the developing arterial walls in human fetuses of different ages suggest that the elastin of the external elastic lamina in the ITA may be laid down by the SMC mass which forms the media, before the formation of the IEL, which would appear to be unusual. Figures 2–20 to 2–25 show developing fetal arteries at the age of 11–12 weeks after conception. It is seen that the ITA and the brachial artery differ from the aorta, common carotid, vertebral, and coronary arteries in regard to the order of development of the internal and external elastic laminae.

This suggests that some degree of orderly arrangement of the medial cells of the arterial wall may occur before the IEL is formed. However, if the IEL is laid down by the SMC of the medial mass first, it is possible that disorganization of these cells may result in errors in the formation of this membrane, particularly with the coronary artery, which is part of the contracting wall of the embryonic heart. Figure 2–26 shows an example of the rather disorganized media of a coronary artery at 15 weeks, with apparent errors in the formation of the IEL.

Other elastic arteries, such as the aorta and carotid, have in common with the ITA multiple layers of elastin in the arterial wall. However, despite these layers of elastin, these arteries show late development of the external elastic lamina and defects in the formation of the IEL; sometimes there are extensive areas of defective formation of this lamina (Fig. 2–27). Uncontrolled growth of

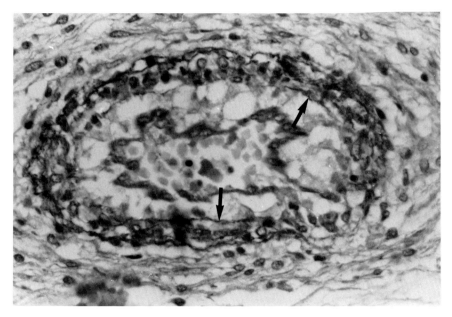

FIGURE 2–21 Section of the wall of the brachial artery at approximately 11 weeks gestation. The EEL is well formed, and the formation of the IEL (arrows) is beginning. The endothelial lining is detached. Orcein-Hx, 500×.

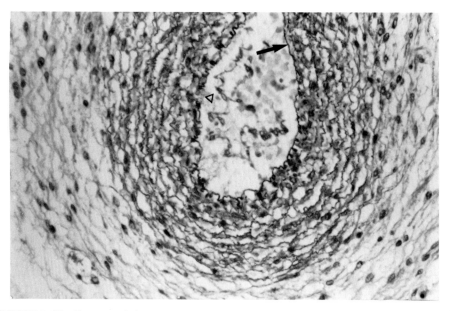

FIGURE 2–22 Section of the aortic wall at 11 weeks gestation. The IEL appears well formed in some areas (arrows), but discontinuities can be seen (arrowhead). There is no defined EEL, but multiple lamellae of elastin are present in the media. The endothelium is detached. Orcein-Hx, 300×.

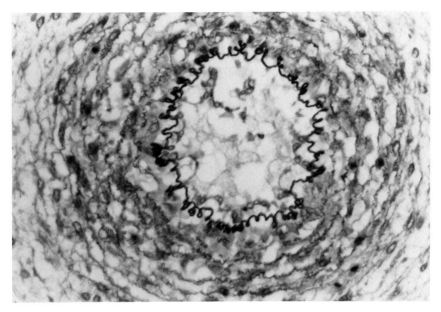

FIGURE 2–23 Section of the common carotid artery at 11 weeks gestation. There is a well-formed IEL and multiple fine lamellae of elastin in the media. Orcein-Hx, 500×.

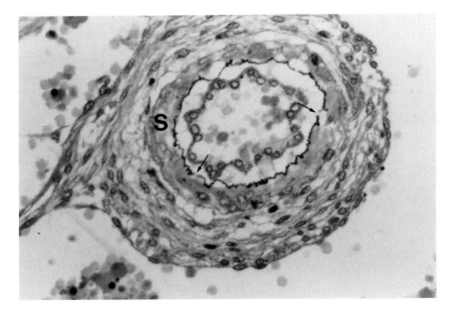

FIGURE 2–24 Section of the vertebral artery at 11 weeks gestation. The media is composed of embryonic SMC (S), with an IEL which is well formed in most areas but appears to contain gaps (arrows). Orcein-Hx, 500×.

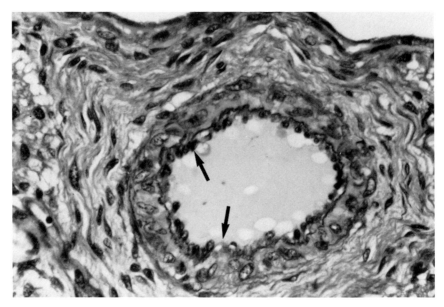

FIGURE 2–25 Section of a coronary artery at 11 weeks gestation. The SMC of the media appear disorganized, and the IEL appears to show discontinuities (arrows) Orcein-Hx, 500×.

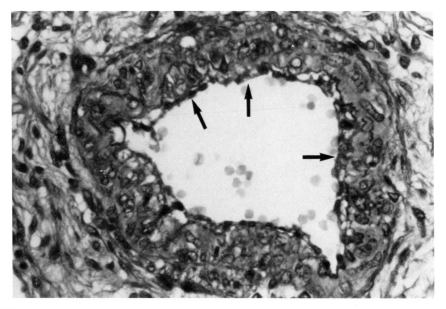

FIGURE 2–26 Section of a coronary artery at 15–16 weeks gestation. The medial SMC appear disorganized, and the IEL appears to be imperfectly formed (arrows). Orcein-Hx, 500×.

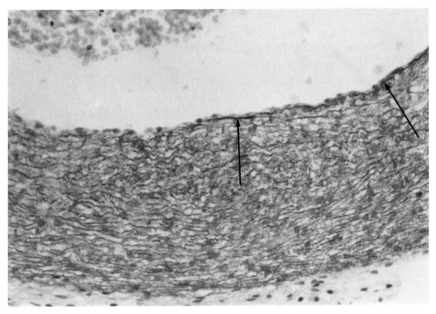

FIGURE 2–27 Cross-section of the aortic wall at 15–16 weeks gestation. The IEL (arrows) is fragmented, with substantial gaps. The media contains large numbers of parallel lamellae of elastin. Orcein-Hx, 300×.

medial SMC in these areas appears inevitable, resulting in significant intimal thickening at birth and in the early years of life. It therefore seems unlikely that multiple layers of elastin in the arterial wall alone ensure proper formation of the IEL.

CONTRIBUTION OF THE ITA TO UNDERSTANDING OF THE DEVELOPMENT OF HUMAN ATHEROSCLEROSIS

The Response to Injury Hypothesis

Comparison of the aging process in the atherosclerosis-prone human coronary artery with that of the relatively immune ITA has proved of great value in the study of human atherosclerosis.

The concept of the initiation of atherosclerotic lesions which is most widely held at present is the "response to injury" hypothesis,[8] in which damaged endothelial cells (caused perhaps by the hemodynamic effects of the circulating blood), platelets, monocytes/macrophages, and SMC may produce growth-stimulating substances which promote proliferation of the medial SMC of the arterial wall.

This concept faces a number of difficulties, particularly the following:

1. Intimal thickening may occur before birth, and the rate of increase of intimal thickening during the first 6 months of life is much greater than during subsequent years.

2. Some human arteries are less affected than others, and a few, such as the ITA, are almost entirely spared.

3. Naturally occurring atherosclerosis is uncommon and slight in extent in many animal species.

4. Atherosclerotic lesions tend to be localized along the length of arteries and around the periphery of the lumen.

5. In experimental animals, superficial endothelial damage alone does not initiate SMC proliferation,[9] and in extensive, prolonged denudation of the inner arterial surface, continued SMC proliferation does not occur.[10]

Intimal thickening has long been considered the most important component in the development of atherosclerosis, and the magnitude of intimal thickening of the coronary arteries appears to be related to the risk of death from coronary insufficiency.[11] Although a local factor associated with the arterial wall has long been suspected[12,13] of being a primary cause of intimal thickening, it has not been clear what this factor might be. The response to injury hypothesis has sought to supply this local component.

Recent Work on the Properties of Vascular Smooth Muscle Cells

The origin of the cells of the thickened arterial intima from medial SMC has been known for some 20 years.[14] More recently, it has become clear that vascular SMC display a range of phenotypes. The two extremes are the "contractile" type, characterized by large cells with numerous microfilament bundles and a low rate of cell division and the "synthetic" type, marked by small cells with very few microfilaments, associated with a relative absence of contractile properties and rapid cell division.[15,16] Such synthetic vascular SMC are found in fetal tissues and neonates. In experimental animals, they mature into the typical contractile type during the first few months after birth.[17] Damage to the vessel wall is associated with modulation of the contractile SMC into the synthetic type, with cell proliferation and the laying down of elastin and collagen in the surrounding matrix.[18,19] Synthetic SMC have been shown to be more active in the synthesis of collagen, elastin, and the proteoglycans of the matrix than the contractile type.[15]

Regulation of the growth of vascular SMC, their phenotype, and their response to contracting and relaxing influences have been the subject of a huge expansion of research in recent years. It has been shown that there is a very complex interaction between endothelium, SMC, and matrix, as well as with growth factors from blood platelets and formed elements of the circulating blood such as monocytes, lymphocytes, and neutrophils.[20-26] A detailed discussion of this aspect and of the pharmacological response of vascular SMC is beyond the limits of this chapter, but a number of recent reviews have been published.[27-31] Much of this work has been carried out on SMC of animal arteries, often in cell culture, and the application of the results to the events of the arterial wall in humans may require further clarification.

The present section describes observations of the arterial walls of humans

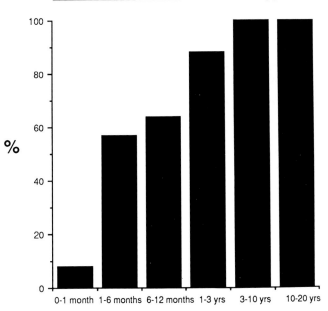

FIGURE 2-28 Mean intimal thickness of the anterior descending coronary artery for age groups 0–20 years. The bar graph shows the percentage of subjects in each age group with intimal thickness (r = mean thickness of intima/thickness of media) greater than 0.1

by light and electron microscopy. By comparing one vessel with another from the same subject, particularly using the ITA as a nearly perfect control, investigators hope to narrow the field and make it easier to approach the most probable sequences of events in the development and progression of human atherosclerosis. The underlying assumption of this approach is that the endothelial cells and SMC present in the walls of different arteries of comparable size from the same subject have essentially the same properties. Recently, differences have been found in the pharmacological response in vitro of the wall of the saphenous vein compared with the ITA.[32,33] The significance of this finding in relation to the use of venous bypass grafts is not yet clear. At present, the major problem with venous arterial grafts appears to arise from rapid intimal thickening by multiplication of medial SMC and edema of the graft wall.

Intimal Thickening in the Human Coronary Artery

Examination of the coronary artery wall in newborn humans shows that in some 8% of cases, intimal thickening of this vessel begins before birth (Fig. 2–28). The rate of increase of intimal thickening in the first 6 months of life, however, is dramatic, and all individuals have significant intimal thickening of these arteries by the age of 3 years. Figure 2–29 shows the mean intimal thickening of the anterior descending coronary artery of various age groups

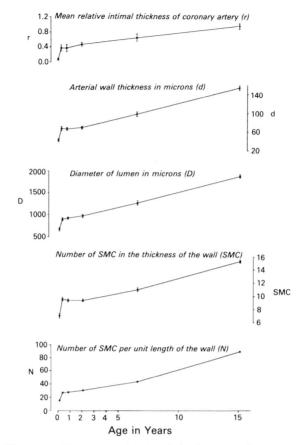

FIGURE 2–29 The rate of increase of intimal thickness with age computed with the rate of growth of SMC in the wall of the anterior descending coronary artery.

and demonstrates that the rate of increase of intimal thickening in the first 6 months is some 20 times that occurring in subsequent years. Figures 2–9, 2–30, and 2–31 illustrate intimal thickening of coronary arteries at the ages of 2 months, 4 months, and 2 years, respectively.

The rapid increase in intimal thickening in the first 6 months parallels the rate of increase in the luminal diameter, the thickenss of the arterial wall, and the number of SMC in the media. It corresponds to the period of rapid growth and adjustment to the circulatory changes which occurs after birth. In uterine life, both ventricules operate in parallel to discharge blood into the systemic circulation, but immediately after birth, they begin to operate in series, and each must pump all of the circulating blood volume. In the case of the left ventricle, this increased activity is performed against a rising systemic blood pressure.[34]

During this period of rapid growth, SMC grow through gaps in the IEL to populate the intima. Although these discontinuities are no more than potential in many subjects at the time of birth, they are readily seen in sections examined by electron microscopy (Fig. 2–32). During the rapid growth of the arterial wall, these potential gaps appear to open and allow penetration by

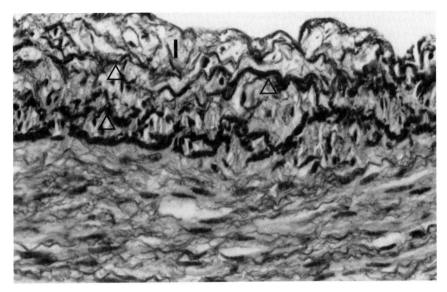

FIGURE 2-30 Transverse section of the coronary artery of a male infant aged 4 months. There are many discontinuities of the IEL, as well as the attempted formation of several imperfect reduplicated IELs (arrowheads). The intima (I) shows marked thickening. Orcein-Hx, 350×.

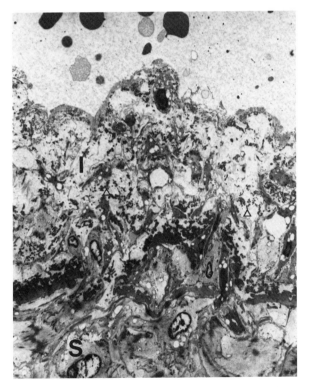

FIGURE 2-31 TEM of thickened intima of the coronary artery of a male child aged 2 years. There are SMC penetrating the gaps in the IEL and scattered, longitudinally oriented elastin fibers (seen here in cross-section—arrowheads) in the intima (I), which is edematous. Medial SMC (S) are also shown. Red blood cells are present in the lumen. Orcein, uranyl acetate, lead citrate, 1,000×.

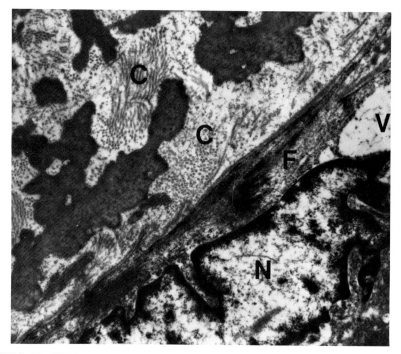

FIGURE 2–32 TEM of the coronary artery of a newborn infant showing a gap in the fragmented IEL (the elastin is stained darkly with orcein). N = nucleus; F = myofibrils; V = vacuole of a medial SMC; C = irregularly arranged collagen fibers in the gap of the IEL. There is no evidence of penetration of the gap by SMC in the plane of this section. Orcein, uranyl acetate, lead citrate 12,000×.

the proliferating SMC of the media to create the musculoelastic zone of the intimal compartment. This vigorous growth response of the SMC of the arterial wall in the first 6 months of life may reflect the immaturity of these cells at the time of birth and their increased growth potential in the "synthetic" form.

The IEL of the ITA, on the other hand, is very well formed at birth, with only tiny gaps apparently too small for penetration by SMC (Fig. 2–3). Although it also develops rapidly, is subjected to rising systemic blood pressure, and has immature SMC, no significant discontinuities develop in the IEL of this vessel in younger age groups (Fig. 2–14), and no intimal thickening occurs.

It thus appears that the initiation of intimal thickening is associated with the presence of discontinuities of the IEL. When such gaps are present, proliferation of SMC into the intimal compartment occurs at a rate dependent on the magnitude of the defects in the IEL and the growth response of these cells.

The Stimulus to Growth of the Medial SMC

It has been established by many in vitro experiments that SMC respond to stretching forces by increased metabolism and realignment in a direction perpendicular to the direction of the stress.[35-39] It is therefore possible that the mechanical stress of the medial SMC at points where the IEL is defective is one of the stimuli to SMC proliferation. Glagov and others[1,2] have shown that the IEL performs an important function in distributing the stresses imposed on the arterial wall by the blood pressure, a function which is disturbed in areas where this membrane is deficient.

Another probable function of the IEL is as a barrier to the diffusion of macromolecules from the circulating plasma into the arterial wall.[40,41] Defects of the IEL would allow infiltration of the media by components of the plasma which may also stimulate the SMC to proliferate. Figures 2–33 and 2–34 show the diffusion of albumin from the arterial lumen outward in the ITA and coronary arteries, respectively.

Some insight into the biological function of the proliferating SMC may be gained by observations of their behavior. These cells form elastin, which initially is laid down in the form of a more or less coherent, reduplicated IEL. This appears to strengthen the arterial wall and repair the defects of the IEL (Figs. 2–7 and 2–9). Sometimes the formation of a reduplicated IEL is relatively effective. For a time, there is no further penetration of this layer by SMC and continued intimal proliferation[41] (Fig. 2–35). In humans, however, this stage is (with the coronary artery particularly) only transient, and breaks occur in the reduplicated IEL associated with further proliferation of SMC. Over time and with multiple cell divisions, elastin production by the proliferating SMC appears to diminish,[42,43] and no coherent sealing membrane on the luminal surface appears to be formed by the cells, which produce variable amounts of discontinuous, longitudinally oriented elastin fibers (Fig. 2–36). Such cells continue to be surrounded by plasma and exposed to the pulsatile stresses of the arterial wall. They may therefore continue to respond to the stimulus to proliferate. This may explain why, in humans, intimal thickening continues to increase at varying rates throughout life.[44]

Coronary Arteries of Domestic Animals

In contrast to humans, naturally occurring atherosclerosis in domestic animals is rare and is slight in extent.[45-49] Figure 2-37 shows the magnitude of the intimal thickening of the anterior descending coronary arteries of young adults of nine different species, compared with that of humans, and Fig. 2-38 shows sections of coronary arteries from the dog, pig, sheep, and baboon.

Examination of the coronary artery structure of these animals shows that the intima, media, and adventitia are essentially the same as those of humans but that they differ in one important respect. The IEL of these vessels is much better formed than that of humans,[50] and in the young animal no significant discontinuities showing the penetration of SMC can be seen and no thickened intima occurs. In some cases, traces of an earlier defective IEL are present, but these have been effectively covered by a substantial reduplicated IEL showing no further discontinuities.

It thus appears that humans are unique among these species in their failure to maintain an effective, coherent IEL in the coronary arteries, although such a well-formed IEL is usually found in the human ITA.

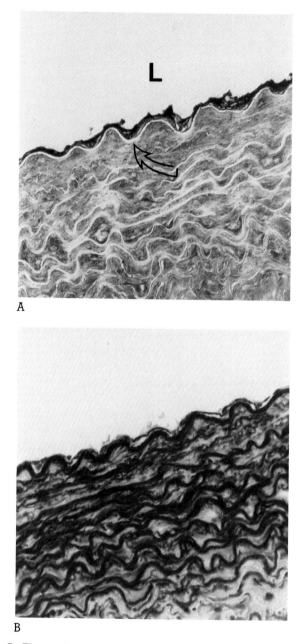

A

B

FIGURE 2-33 **A:** The wall of the ITA of a male child aged 3 years, stained by the immunoperoxidase technique for albumin. The artery is normal in structure and shows the abrupt decline of albumin concentration at the luminal face of the IEL (arrow). The elastin does not admit molecules the size of albumin, and the intact IEL appears to form an effective barrier to diffusion of albumin from the lumen (L). 350×. **B:** The same artery (a sequential section) stained with orcein-Hx. There is a normal intima, which occupies the area uniformly infiltrated by albumin. 350×.

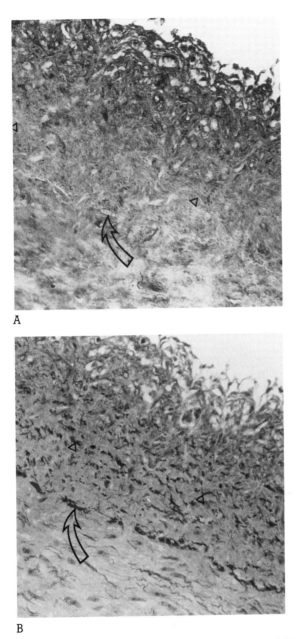

A

B

FIGURE 2–34 A: The wall of a coronary artery from a male aged 19 years. Albumin stain 350×. The figure shows the fragmented, unstained elastin of the IEL containing several gaps (large arrow) and further unstained elastin in the thickened intima (arrowheads). 350×. **B:** The same arterial wall (sequential section) stained with orcein-Hx, 350×. The gaps in the fragmented IEL are shown (large arrow), as well as the unsuccessful formation of reduplicated IELs (arrowheads), with a progressive decline of elastin deposition toward the lumen. No formed barrier layer is present at the luminal margin of the thickened intima.

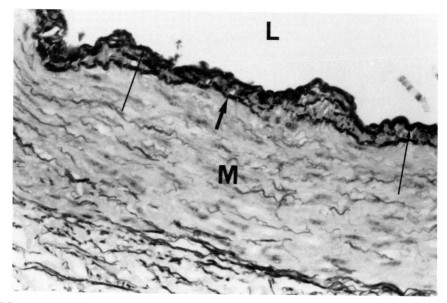

FIGURE 2–35 The anterior descending coronary artery of a male aged 18 years. There is an unusually well-formed, reduplicated IEL (small arrows) showing no discontinuities on the luminal side of the original IEL (large arrow). Intimal thickening ($r = 0.15$) and the proportion of discontinuities of the IEL (12%) were less than average for the age group (0.97 and 23.8, respectively). L = lumen; M = media. Orcein-Hx, $200 \times$.

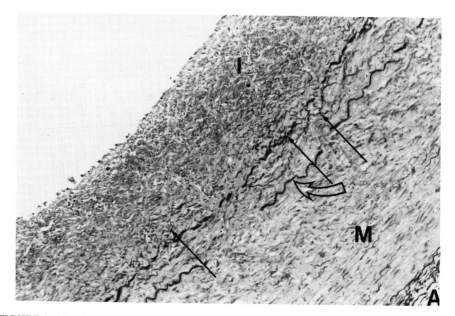

FIGURE 2–36 Coronary artery of a male aged 48 years. There is substantial intimal thickening, with deficiencies of the original IELs (large arrow). Imperfectly formed, reduplicated IELs (small arrows) are present. Elastin formation by the SMC of the intima declines toward the lumen. I = intima; M = media; A = adventitia.

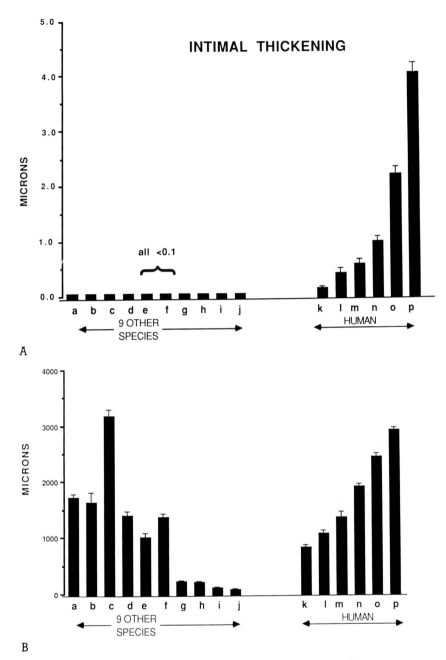

FIGURE 2–37 A: Intimal thickening of the left anterior descending coronary artery of nine different species compared with humans. The ages of the various groups in years are in brackets. (a) Pigs (8/12), (b) cattle (6/12–1), (c) cattle (1 1/2–2), (d) sheep (1), (e) dogs (3–5), (f) baboons (1 1/2), (g) rabbits (8/12), (h) chickens (7–8/12), (i) rats (8/12–1), (j) mice (6–8/12), (k) to (p) humans, ages (0–1), (1–3), (3–10), 10–20), (20–40), (40–60). **B:** Mean diameter of the lumen of the coronary arteries from the same species, showing that in six of them, the size of the vessels is comparable to that of human coronary arteries.

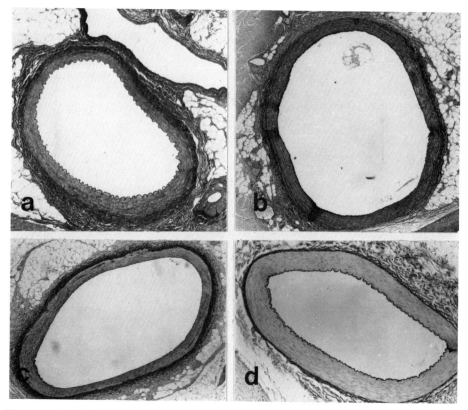

FIGURE 2–38 Transverse sections of anterior descending coronary arteries of (**A**) dog (36×), (**B**) swine (19×), (**C**) sheep (27×), and (**D**) baboon (19×). There is insignificant intimal thickening of these vessels. Orcein-Hx.

Other Evidence Indicating the Importance of the IEL in the Development of Intimal Thickening

The repair reaction of the medial SMC to defects of the IEL is seen in many different circumstances in experimental animals, as well as in human subjects.

1. When the elastin of the arterial wall is damaged by irradiation in the experimental animal, intimal thickening similar in histological structure to naturally occurring intimal thickening in humans occurs.[51,52] (Fig. 2–39).

2. If the IEL is damaged by trauma, such as in various types of balloon injury, intimal thickening occurs[53,54] (Fig. 2–40). However, superficial injury, involving only the endothelial surface, does not incite such a proliferative response.[9]

3. The normal formation of elastin depends on copper-containing enzymes which play an essential role in the cross-linking of elastin molecules. This is a critical factor in the mechanical properties of this substance

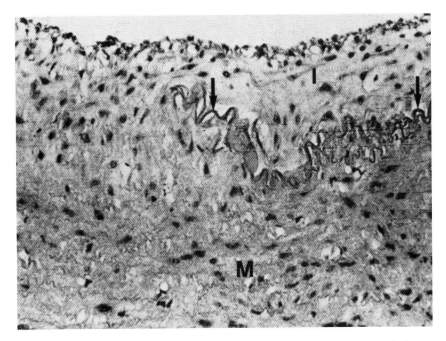

FIGURE 2–39 Transverse section of the aortic wall of a rabbit which has been exposed to x-radiation. There is destruction of the IEL (arrows), with growth of medial cells into the intimal compartment. M = media; I = intima. (From Lindsay S, et al: Aortic atherosclerosis in the dog after localized aortic X-irradiation. *Circ Res* 10:51–60, 1962. Reproduced by permission of the American Heart Association, Inc., and the author.)

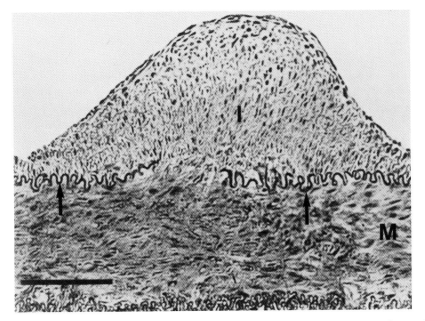

FIGURE 2–40 Transverse section of a rabbit aorta which has been subjected to baloon injury. There is damage to the IEL (arrows) and growth of medial cells producing gross intimal thickening. I = intima; M = media. (From Bjorkerud S: Atherosclerosis initiated by mechanical trauma in normolipidaemic rabbits. *J Atheroscl Res* 9:209–213, 1969. Reproduced by permission of Elsevier Science Publishers and the author.)

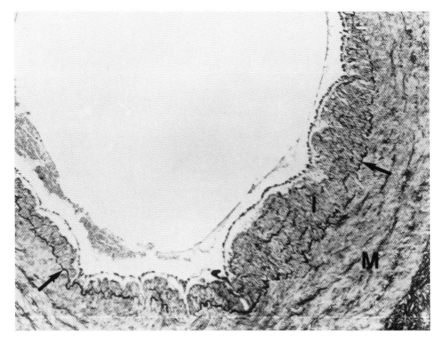

FIGURE 2–41 Transverse section of the coronary artery of a copper-deficient pig. There is fragmentation of the IEL (arrow), with growth of SMC through the defects causing pronounced intimal thickening. I = intima; M = media. (From Coulson WF, et al: Cardiovascular studies on copper deficient swine. V. The histogenesis of the coronary artery lesions. *Am J Pathol* 43:945–954, 1963. Reproduced by permission of the *American Journal of Pathology*.)

and its ability to allow stretching and deformation, with return to its original size and shape. In copper-deficient swine, elastin is imperfectly formed; the IEL of these arteries shows discontinuities and intimal thickening[55] (Fig. 2–41). A genetic disorder of humans (Menkes' syndrome) is due to defective absorption of copper. Infants with this syndrome also show imperfect elastin formation and disruption of the IEL, with early intimal thickening. Most of them die before the age of 3 years from the resulting complications[56] (Fig. 2–42).

4. When the arterial wall of humans is involved in an inflammatory reaction, discontinuities of the IEL develop, perhaps due to elastases and collagenases produced by the inflammatory cells. Under these circumstances, intimal thickening due to the proliferation of medial cells into the intimal compartment occurs even in small arteries which normally do not suffer intimal thickening[6,41] (Fig. 2–43).

5. The same type of intimal thickening of small arteries is seen in the vicinity of the tumor cells in malignant disease, where the damage to the IEL may result from enzymes produced by the neoplastic cells or by the inflammatory cells surrounding the tumor deposit[57] (Fig. 2–44).

6. The human aorta does not have an intact IEL, and intimal thickening begins in areas where this is poorly formed. Figure 2–45–C shows the

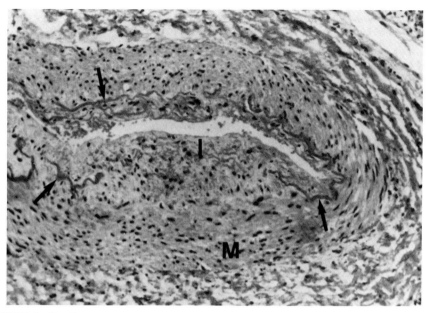

FIGURE 2–42 Transverse section of the coronary artery of a human infant with Menkes' syndrome. There is disorganization of the IEL (arrows) showing gross discontinuities with growth of medial cells into the intimal compartment. I = intima; M = media; A = adventitia. (From Danks DM, et al: Menkes' kinky hair syndrome: An inherited defect in copper absorption with widespread effects. *Pediatrics* 50:188–201, 1972. Reproduced by permission of *Pediatrics*.)

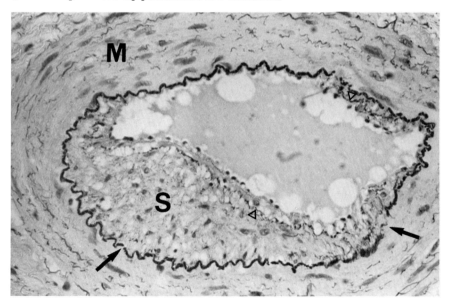

FIGURE 2–43 Intimal thickening of a small artery involved in an inflammatory reaction showing SMC (S) populating the intima through defects in the IEL (arrows). Imperfectly formed, reduplicated IELs have been formed by the proliferating SMC (arrowheads). M = media. Orcein-Hx, 300×.

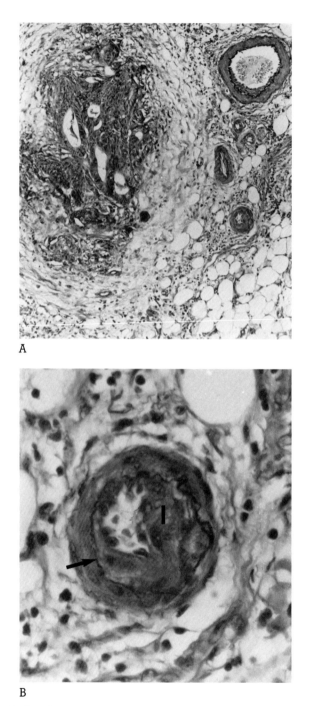

A

B

FIGURE 2–44   **A:** Small arteries in the vicinity of a metastatic deposit of carcinoma of the colon. Verhoeff's Elastin van Gieson (EVG), 80×. **B:** Higher-power view of one of the small arteries in (A) showing disorganization and discontinuities of the IEL (arrow) and pronounced intimal thickening (I), with narrowing of the lumen. Verhoeff's EVG, 450×.

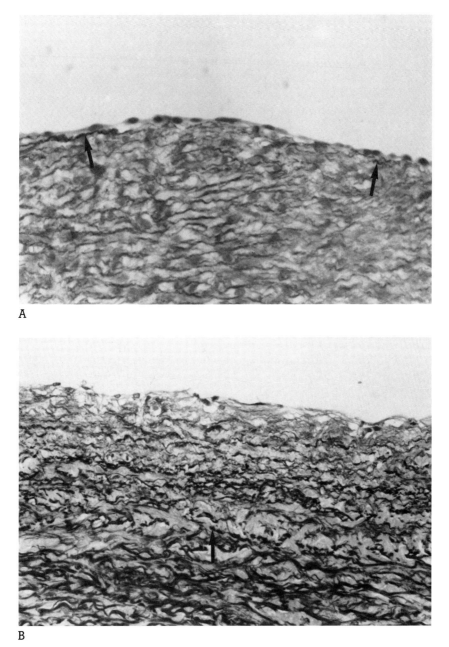

A

B

FIGURE 2–45 A: Aortic wall in an 11-week-old fetus. The IEL (arrows) shows a defect, with incipient intimal thickening due to the growth of medial SMC through this area. Orcein-Hx, 500×. **B:** Aortic wall of a male aged 23 years. There is substantial intimal thickening. The arrow shows the position of the original IEL. Orcein-Hx, 200×.

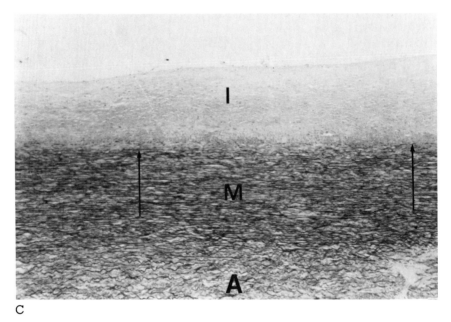

C

FIGURE 2–45 Continued C: Aortic wall of a female aged 58 years from an area apparently normal by naked eye examination. There is gross intimal thickening (I) and a discontinuous IEL (arrows). M = media; A = adventitia. Orcein-Hx 50×.

aortic wall at 11 weeks, 23 years, and 58 years, respectively. Similarly, other elastic arteries such as the common carotid, which may have a better-formed IEL, present deficiencies of this membrane especially in older age groups, and intimal thickening develops. Similar deficiencies of the IEL are present in medium-sized (muscular) arteries and are associated with intimal thickening (Figs. 2–9 to 2–11). Arteries such as the radial and tibial have been shown to be slower in developing arterial disease, and these have a better-formed IEL than the coronary arteries or the great vessels mentioned.[58,59]

7. Although large veins develop slight intimal thickening with age (Fig. 2–46), when they are inserted into the arterial system and subjected to pulsatile arterial pressure, as in bypass surgery, intimal thickening develops rapidly, often resulting in serious narrowing of the lumen. This intimal thickening arises in the same way as in arteries, by the growth of medial SMC through defects in the IEL into the intimal compartment[60-62] (Fig. 2–47).

8. There is an enhanced rate of intimal thickening in the major arteries in arterial hypertension[63-67] and in the pulmonary arteries in pulmonary hypertension,[68,69] indicating that increased intra-arterial pressure may result in increased stimulation of SMC to grow through defects in the arterial wall. It is possible that the enhanced pressure may increase the

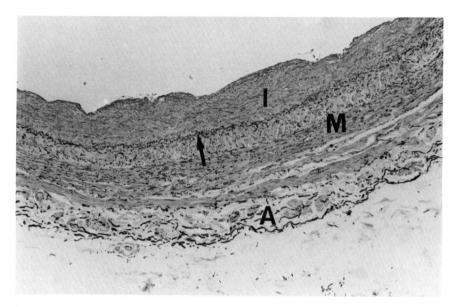

FIGURE 2-46 Saphenous vein from an older patient prepared for use as a graft. I = thickened intima; M = media; A = adventitia; arrow = imperfectly formed IEL. 80×.

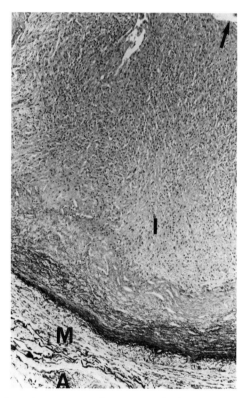

FIGURE 2-47 Failed saphenous vein bypass graft showing gross intimal thickening from proliferation of medial SMC. I = intima; M = media; A = adventitia. The arrow indicates the lumen.

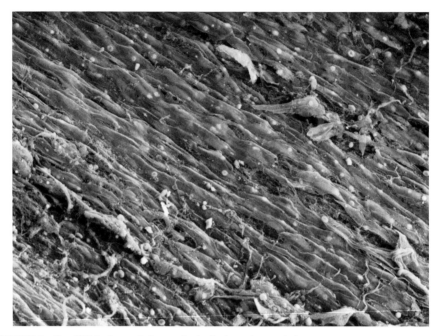

FIGURE 2-48 SEM view of the endothelial surface of the coronary artery of a male aged 18 years. It shows detachment of endothelial cells, with many bare areas. 360×.

magnitude of the discontinuities in the IEL, which would also tend to increase the rate of intimal thickening.

Complications of Intimal Thickening

Intimal thickening has been well established as an integral part of the aging process in humans, and at an earlier stage in the study of atherosclerosis it was accepted as normal,[70] especially in the first years of life. The process of intimal thickening merges, however, without any line of demarcation, into the full picture of atherosclerosis. Evidence already presented shows that the magnitude of intimal thickening correlates with death from coronary artery insufficiency,[11] and from the study of the ITA, there is strong evidence that in the absence of intimal thickening, there is no atherosclerosis.

The luminal surface of the ITA in younger age groups is completely covered by regularly arranged endothelial cells (Fig. 2–4). This, however, is not the case with the coronary arteries in the presence of substantial intimal thickening[71] (Figs. 2–48 to 2–50). The firm attachment of the endothelial cells may depend on proximity to a coherent underlying elastin membrane, which in general is absent in the presence of pronounced intimal thickening (Figs. 2–51 and 2–52). Due to the loose, edematous nature of the thickened intima and

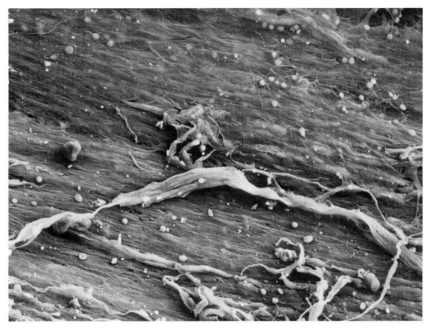

FIGURE 2–49 SEM view of the luminal surface of the coronary artery of a male aged 59 years. There is total loss of endothelial cells in this area, which shows scattered, adherent red blood cells and leukocytes. No significant deposition of activated platelets or fibrin is present. 365×.

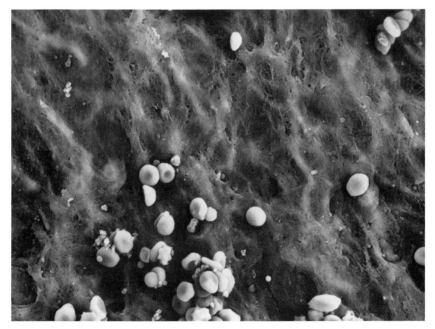

FIGURE 2–50 The bare area (SEM) from the coronary artery of a male aged 32 years. There are adherent red blood cells and a few scattered platelets, but no substantial covering of the area by platelets or fibrin. 1,070×.

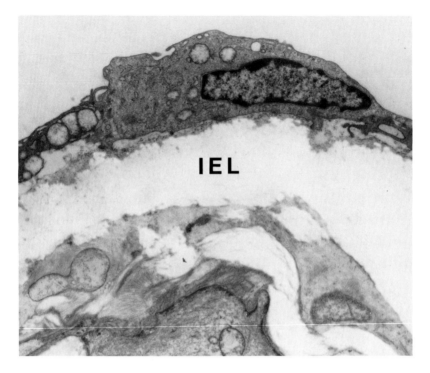

FIGURE 2-51 TEM section of the ITA of a male child aged 2 years. The endothelial cell is in close relationship with the IEL (unstained) and is apparently attached to it by microfibrils. Uranyl acetate and lead citrate, 8,000×.

the disorganized elastin deposits, the anchorage of endothelial cells in this situation appears to be precarious (Fig. 2–53), and extensive bare areas are present on the luminal surface. These bare areas show no evidence of significant platelet or fibrin covering.

Under these conditions, there is no barrier to the free entry to the edematous intima of formed elements of the circulating blood such as red blood cells, leukocytes, and macrophages. In addition, there is unobstructed entry to the intima of macromolecules of all sizes, including lipoproteins. It has been calculated[54] that the rate of influx of lipoprotein to the intima in animal experiments is 15 times as great through bare areas. Such complications may be expected to increase the rate of intimal thickening, and account for the presence of foamy macrophages and lipid deposits in the intima (Fig. 2–54), since the influx of lipid may exceed the capacity of the intimal cells to metabolize this material.

It thus appears that once intimal thickening has begun, further progression of this process with time in the larger vessels of humans is inevitable. The rate of increase of intimal thickness depends on a number of factors associated with the smooth muscle cells themselves—their capacity for growth, their

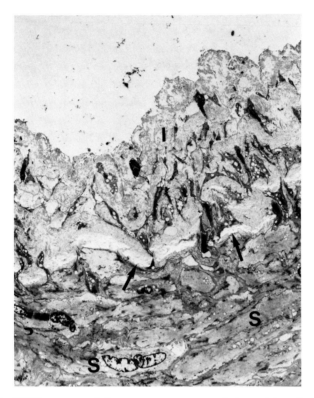

FIGURE 2-52 TEM section of the coronary artery of the subject in Figs 2-31 and 2-51 showing the disorganized IEL (unstained-arrows) and the thickened intima (I), which is edematous and not covered by endothelial cells on its luminal surface. S = smooth muscle cells of the media. 1,000×.

ability to synthesize elastin and form an effective sealing layer on the luminal surface, and the degree of edema of the thickened intima. The rate of increase also depends on the influx of the thickened intima of red blood cells, leukocytes, macrophages, and lipoproteins.

The absence of significant intimal thickening in normal smaller arteries may be due to several factors. These vessels may have a better-formed IEL, and they are subjected to a lower blood pressure, with a smaller pulsatile component. They have, however, the capacity to develop intimal thickening if their IEL is damaged and if there is an increase in luminal pressure, as occurs in the inflammation[6,41] or in the vicinity of active tumor growth.[57] After the disappearance of the damaging influence, they have greater ability to re-form an effective sealing inner lining or a reduplicated IEL, and they may not show such progressive intimal thickening as that of the major arteries.

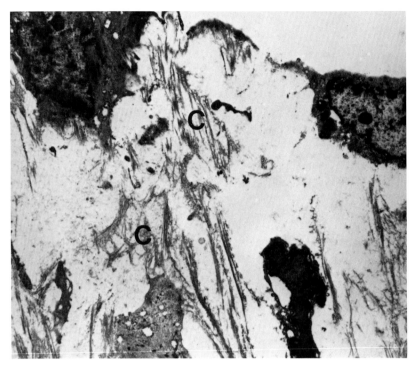

FIGURE 2–53 TEM section from the coronary artery of a male aged 59 years. The section is from an area which still has endothelial cells present on the luminal surface. It shows the precarious attachment of these cells to scanty collagen fibers (C) of the edematous, thickened intima. 3,500×.

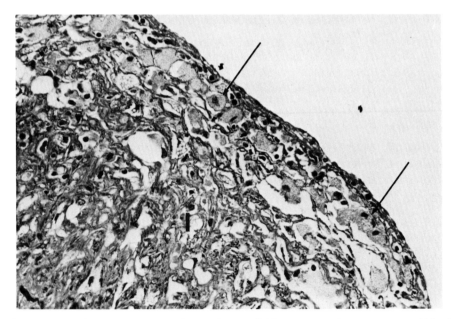

FIGURE 2–54 Coronary artery of a male aged 19 years, with gross intimal thickening. The intima contains large numbers of foamy macrophages (arrows) and leukocytes in the disorganized stroma. Orcein-Hx, 400×.

REFERENCES

1. Glagov S, Wolinsky H: Aortic wall as a "two phase" material. *Nature* 199:606–608, 1963.
2. Wolinsky H, Glagov S: Structural basis for the static mechanical properties of the aortic media. *Circ Res* 14:400–413, 1964.
3. Burton AC: Relation of structure to function of the tissues of the wall of blood vessels. *Physiol Rev* 34:619–642, 1954.
4. Cliff WJ: *Blood Vessels*. Cambridge, Cambridge University Press, 1976.
5. Ross R, Glomsett JA: The pathogenesis of atherosclerosis. *N Engl J med* 295:369–377, 420–425, 1976.
6. Sims FH: Discontinuities in the internal elastic lamina: A comparison of coronary and internal mammary arteries. *Artery* 13:127–143, 1985.
7. Lansing AI: Elastic tissue. In *The Arterial Wall*. Baltimore, Williams & Wilkins Co., 1959, p 136.
8. Ross R: The pathogenesis of atherosclerosis—an update. *N Engl J Med* 314:488–500, 1986.
9. Reidy MA, Schwartz SM: Endothelial regeneration. III. Time course of intimal changes after small defined injury to rat aortic endothelium. *Lab Invest* 44:301–308, 1981.
10. Clowes AW, Clowes MM, Reidy MA: Kinetics of cellular proliferation after arterial injury III. Endothelial and smooth muscle growth in chronically denuded vessels. *Lab Invest* 54:295–303, 1986.
11. Sims FH: A comparison of coronary and internal mammary arteries, and implications of the results in the etiology of atherosclerosis. *Am Heart J* 105:560–566, 1983.
12. Dock W: The predilection of atherosclerosis for the coronary arteries. *JAMA* 131:875–878, 1946.
13. Gillman T: Reduplication, remodeling, regeneration, repair, and degeneration of arterial elastic membranes. Some implications for the pathogenesis of arterial diseases. *Arch Pathol* 67:624–642, 1959.
14. Hassler O: The origin of the cells constituting arterial intima thickening. An experimental autoradiographic study with the use of H3-thymidine. *Lab Invest* 22:286–293, 1970.
15. Campbell GR, Campbell JH, Manderson JA, et al: Arterial smooth muscle. A multifunctional mesenchymal cell. *Arch Pathol Lab Med* 112:977–986, 1988.
16. Dilley RJ, McGeachie JK, Prendergast FJ: A review of the proliferative behaviour, morphology, and phenotypes of vascular smooth muscle. *Atherosclerosis* 63:99–107, 1987.
17. Nikkari ST, Rantala I, Pystynen P, et al: Characterisation of the phenotype of smooth muscle cells in human fetal aorta on the basis of ultrastructure, immunofluorescence, and the composition of cytoskeletal and cytocontractile proteins. *Atherosclerosis* 74:33–40, 1988.
18. Gabbiani G, Kocher O, Bloom WS, et al: Actin expression in smooth muscle cells of rat aortic intimal thickening, human atheromatous plaque, and cultured rat aortic media. *J Clin Invest* 73:148–152, 1984.
19. Kocher O, Skalli I, Bloom WS, et al: Cytoskeleton of rat aortic smooth muscle cells: Normal conditions and experimental intimal thickening. *Lab Invest* 50:645–652, 1984.

20. Campbell JH, Campbell GR: Endothelial cell influences on vascular smooth muscle phenotype. *Annu Rev Physiol* 48:295–306, 1986.

21. Arciniegas E, Pulido M, Pereyra B: Growth response of endothelial and smooth muscle cells to a collagen matrix throughout development. *Atherosclerosis* 73:71–80, 1988.

22. Navab M, Hough GP, Stevenson LW, et al: Monocyte migration into the subendothelial space of a co-culture of adult human aortic endothelial and smooth muscle cells. *J Clin Invest* 82:1853–1863, 1988.

23. Prescott MF, McBride CK, Court M: Development of intimal lesions after leucocyte migration into the vascular wall. *Am J Pathol* 135:835–846, 1989.

24. Rennick RE, Campbell JH, Campbell GR: Vascular smooth muscle phenotype and growth behaviour can be influenced by macrophages in vitro. *Atherosclerosis* 71:35–43, 1988.

25. Koo EWY, Gottlieb AI: Kinetics of cellular proliferation after arterial injury. V. Role of acute distension in the induction of smooth muscle proliferation. *Am J Pathol* 134:497–503, 1989.

26. Nomoto A, Mutoh S, Hagihara H, et al: Smooth muscle cell migration induced by inflammatory cells products, and its inhibition by a potent calcium antagonist, nilvadipine. *Atherosclerosis* 72:213–219, 1988.

27. Dzau VJ, Gibbons GH: Cell biology of vascular hypertrophy in systemic hypertension. *Am J Cardiol* 62:30G–35G, 1988.

28. Waldman SA, Murad F: Biochemical mechanisms underlying vascular smooth muscle relaxation: The guanylate cyclase—cyclic GMP system. *J Cardiovasc Pharm* 12(Suppl 5):S115–S118, 1988.

29. Nakatsu K, Diamond J: Role of cyclic GMP in relaxation of vascular and other smooth muscle. *Can J Physiol Pharmacol* 67:251–262, 1989.

30. Pomerantz KB, Hajjar DP: Eicosanoids in the regulation of arterial smooth muscle cell phenotype, proliferating capacity and cholesterol metabolism. *Arteriosclerosis* 9:413–429, 1989.

31. Caramelo C, Okada K, Tsai P, et al: Mechanisms of the vascular effect of pressor hormones. *Am J Cardiol* 62:47G–53G, 1988.

32. Yang Z, Diederich D, Schneider K, et al: Endothelium-derived relaxing factor and protection against contractions induced by histamine and serotonin in the human internal mammary artery and in the saphenous vein. *Circulation* 80:1041–1048, 1989.

33. Chaikhouni A, Crawford FA, Kochel PJ, et al: Human internal mammary artery produces more prostacyclin than saphenous vein. *J Thorac Cardiovasc Surg* 92:88–91, 1986.

34. Beck F, Moffat DB, Davies DP: *Human Embryology*. Oxford, Blackwell Scientific Publications, 1985, pp 213–216.

35. Leung DYM, Glagov S, Mathews MB: Cyclic stretching stimulates synthesis of matrix components by arterial smooth muscle cells in vitro. *Science* 191:475–477, 1976.

36. Merrilees MJ, Merriless MA, Birnbaum PS, et al: The effect of centrifugal force on glycosaminoglycan production by aortic smooth muscle cells in culture. *Atherosclerosis* 27:259–264, 1977.

37. Buck RC: Behaviour of vascular smooth muscle cells during repeated stretching of the substratum in vitro. *Atherosclerosis* 46:217–223, 1983.

38. Sottiurai VS, Kolros P, Glagov S, et al: Morphological alterations of cultured arterial smooth muscle cells by cyclic stretching. *J Surg Res* 35:490–497, 1983.

39. Dartsch PC, Hammerle H, Betz E: Orientation of cultured arterial smooth muscle cells growing on cyclically stretched substrates. *Acta Anat* 125:108–113, 1966

40. Smith EB, Staples EM: Distribution of plasma proteins across the human aortic wall. Barrier functions of endothelium and internal elastic lamina. *Atherosclerosis* 37:579–590, 1980.

41. Sims FH: The internal elastic lamina in normal and abnormal human arteries. A barrier to the diffusion of macromolecules from the lumen. *Artery* 16:159–173, 1989.

42. Campbell GR, Chamley-Campbell JH: Invited review: The cellular pathobiology of atherosclerosis. *Pathology* 13:423–440, 1981.

43. Schwartz SM, Campbell GR, Campbell JH: Replication of smooth muscle cells in vascular disease. *Circ Res* 58:427–444, 1986.

44. Sims FH, Gavin JB: The early development of intimal thickening of human coronary arteries. *Coronary Artery Dis* 1:205–213, 1990

45. Finlayson R, Symons C: Comparative aspects of arterial disease. In Chalmers DG, Gresham GA: (Eds), *Biological Aspects of Occlusive Arterial Disease*. Cambridge, Cambridge University Press, 1964, pp 333–340.

46. Dahme EG: Atherosclerosis and arteriosclerosis in domestic animals. *Ann NY Acad Sci* 127:657–670, 1965.

47. Luginbuhl H, Jones JET: The morphology or morphogenesis of atherosclerosis in aged swine. *Ann NY Acad Sci* 127:763–779, 1965.

48. Gresham GA, Howard AN: Vascular lesions in primates. *Ann NY Acad Sci* 127:694–701, 1965.

49. Gilbert C, Gillman J: Structural modifications in the coronary artery of the baboon (*Papio ursinus*) with special reference to age and endocrine status. *S Afr J Med Sci* 25:59–70, 1960.

50. Sims FH: A comparison of structural features of the walls of coronary arteries from 10 different species. *Pathology* 21:115–124, 1989.

51. Lindsay S, Kohn HI, Dakin R, et al: Aortic atherosclerosis in the dog after localized aortic X-radiation. *Circ Res* 10:51–60, 1962.

52. Lindsay S, Entenman C, Ellis EE, et al: Aortic atherosclerosis in the dog after localized aortic irradiation with electrons. *Circ Res* 10:61–67, 1962.

53. Bjorkerud S: Atherosclerosis initiated by mechanical trauma in normolipidaemic rabbits. *J Atheroscl Res* 9:209–213, 1969.

54. Bondjers G, Bjorkerud S: Arterial repair and atherosclerosis after mechanical injury. Part 3. Cholesterol accumulation and removal in morphologically defined regions of aortic atherosclerotic lesions in the rabbit. *Atherosclerosis* 17:85–94, 1973.

55. Coulson WF, Carnes WH: Cardiovascular studies on copper deficient swine. V. The histogenesis of the coronary artery lesions. *Am J Pathol* 43:945–954, 1963.

56. Danks DM, Campbell PE, Stevens BJ, et al: Menkes' kinky hair syndrome: An inherited defect in copper absorption with widespread effects. *Pediatrics* 50:188–201, 1972.

57. Sims FH: The arterial wall in malignant disease. *Atherosclerosis* 32:445–450, 1979.

58. Sappington SW, Cook HS: Radial artery changes in comparison with those of the coronary and other arteries. *Am J Med Sci* 192:822–839, 1936.

59. Sappington SW, Hornet JA: Tibial artery changes in comparison with those of the radial and coronary arteries. *Am J Med Sci* 201:862–871, 1941.

60. Jones M, Conkle DM, Ferrans VJ, et al: Lesions observed in arterial autogenous vein grafts. Light and electron microscope evaluation. *Circulation* 47(Suppl. III):198–210, 1973.

61. Unni KK, Kottke BA, Titus JL, et al: Pathologic changes in aorto-coronary saphenous vein grafts. *Am J Cardiol* 34:526–532, 1974.

62. Van der Lei B, Wildevuur CRH, Nieuwenhuis P: Compliance and biodegradation of vascular grafts stimulate the regeneration of elastic laminae in neo-arterial tissue: An experimental study in rats. *Surgery* 99:45–52, 1986.

63. Folkow B: Structure and function of the arteries in hypertension. *Am Heart J* 114:938–948, 1987.

64. Grunwald J, Chobanian AV, Haudenschild CC: Smooth muscle cell migration and proliferation: Atherogenic mechanisms in hypertension. *Atherosclerosis* 67:215–221, 1987.

65. Seidel CA, Schildmeyer LA: Vascular smooth muscle adaptation to increased load. *Annu Rev Physiol* 49:489–499, 1987.

66. Gordon D, Schwartz SM: Replication of smooth muscle cells in hypertension and atherosclerosis. *Am J Cardiol* 59:44A–48A, 1987.

67. Schwartz SM, Reidy MA: Common mechanism of proliferation of smooth muscle cells in atherosclerosis and hypertension. *Hum Pathol* 18:240–247, 1987.

68. Easterly JA, Glagov S, Ferguson DJ: Morphogenesis of intimal obliterative hyperplasia of small arteries in experimental pulmonary hypertension. *Am J Pathol* 52:325–347, 1968.

69. Moore GW, Smith RRL, Hutchins GM: Pulmonary artery atherosclerosis. *Arch Pathol Lab Med* 106:378–380, 1982.

70. Haust MD: Atherosclerosis in childhood. *Perspect Pediatr Pathol* 4:155–216, 1978.

71. Sims FH, Gavin JB, Vanderwee MA: The intima of human coronary arteries. *Am Heart J* 118:32–38, 1989.

CHAPTER **3**

Preoperative Evaluation and the Angiographic Anatomy of the Internal Thoracic Arteries

RAM N. SINGH

INTRODUCTION

The internal thoracic arteries (ITAs) have been utilized for myocardial revascularization due to their predictable intrathoracic course and anatomical proximity to the heart. This is particularly true of the left ITA, which, if dissected to the fifth costal cartilage level, conveniently reaches the coronary arteries in the anterolateral surface of the heart. The left ITA can be used almost routinely for this purpose, provided that proximal subclavian atherosclerosis has been ruled out. This has become the most commonly used graft for coronary revascularization.

Excellent long-term results of the ITA grafts published in the mid 1980s have created enthusiasm for bilateral and sequential ITA grafts. For these complex schemes of ITA grafting, longer pedicles are required to reach the posterior coronary circulation. This may necessitate distal dissection to and beyond the terminal bifurcation, where the anatomy and vessel caliber are variable. In these cases, preoperative arteriographic delineation of the ITAs is helpful in planning the surgical procedure.

MATERIALS AND EQUIPMENT

The ITAs can be visualized at the end of a routine left heart catheterization, utilizing the same x-ray equipment used for coronary arteriography. Selective or nearly selective injection of the contrast agent is needed for accurate delin-

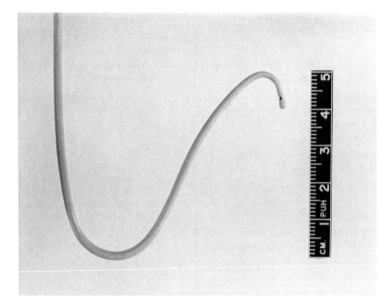

FIGURE 3–1 Brachial internal mammary catheter.

eation of the anatomy. Aortic root or subclavian arteriograms produce unsatisfactory ITA visualization even when digital subtraction techniques are used. Internal thoracic arteriography should be performed, using a 6- or 7-inch image intensifier and recorded on 35mm cine film or a high-quality videotape at 30 frames per second.

CATHETERIZATION TECHNIQUE

Those using Judkin's technique for left heart catheterization may use the femoral internal mammary catheter. Usually the left ITA is easily catheterized with this technique, but the right ITA is difficult to reach, particularly if there is tortuosity of the innominate artery. Further, the commercially available femoral internal mammary catheters are somewhat unsafe, due to their large, stiff tip. Instances of dissection of the ITA orifice and the subclavian artery have been reported.

These technical difficulties prompted the author to develop the technique of visualization of both ITAs using a right brachial approach.[1]

A special preformed brachial internal mammary catheter (Fig. 3–1) is manufactured by the Cordis Corporation of Miami, Florida. The catheter is made of polyurethane, No. 8 French, and is 80 cm long, having two preformed curvatures, the larger, 7.5 cm from the tip and the smaller 1 cm at the tip in the direction opposite to the primary curve. The catheter gently tapers down to a

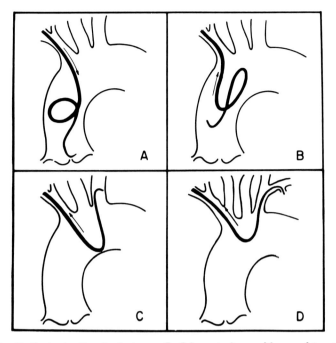

FIGURE 3-2 Catheterization technique. **A:** A loop is formed by pushing the catheter tip against the aortic valve. **B:** The catheter is pulled back. **C:** The large curvature is recovered, and the tip engages the left subclavian artery. **D:** The catheter is pulled back to advance the catheter tip into the left ITA. (From Singh RN: Internal mammary arteriography: A new catheter technique by right brachial approach. *Cathet and Cardiovasc Diagn* 6:439–449, 1980.)

No. 5 1/2 French at the tip, with an open end and two side holes. The inside diameter is uniform to allow a 0.038-inch guide wire.

The brachial internal mammary catheter is introduced via brachial arteriotomy in the right arm. The flexible catheter tip is straightened with the index finger for introduction. No guide wire is usually necessary. As the catheter is advanced to the wider lumen of the subclavian artery, the short preformed tip bends, and the catheter is easily advanced to the aortic root under fluoroscopic control. A loop is formed by pushing the catheter tip against the aortic valve (Fig. 3–2A). A sudden pull of the catheter will recover the primary curve. The tip is now directed toward the left part of the aortic arch (Fig. 3–2B,C). The origin of the left subclavian artery is engaged by torquing and manipulation. At this stage, pulling the catheter will advance the tip in the subclavian artery toward the ITA orifice (Fig. 3–2D). Some manipulation is necessary to engage the tip into the orifice.

The selective injection of radiopaque contrast material into the ITAs produces intense pain. This can be minimized by diluting 76% Renografin with an equal amount of 5% dextrose in water. Injection of 3 to 4 cc of diluted Renografin will produce good opacification. Recently introduced nonionic contrast agents can be used to further minimize the pain.

Using this technique, catheterization of the left ITA can be done in 4 to 5 minutes and good visualization can be obtained in over 90% of cases. The Selective catheterization of the right ITA is performed as the catheter is withdrawn in the right subclavian artery. The catheter tip simply falls into the right ITA orifice when it reaches the first part of the right subclavian artery. Very little manipulation is necessary. The right ITA can be visualized 100% of the time using this catheter in less than a minute.

RADIOGRAPHIC TECHNIQUE

Internal thoracic arteriograms are best recorded in posteroanterior projection, keeping the image intensifier in close contact with the patient's chest. From their origin, the ITAs are covered by "panning" in their entire intrathoracic course. Shallow oblique views may be used to separate the distal ITA image from the paraspinal density.

ESTIMATION OF THE ITA's DIAMETER

Arteriograms are viewed on a 35mm cine projector. The magnification factor is determined by dividing the known diameter of the catheter tip (1.8 mm) by the measured diameter of its image on the viewing screen. The luminal diameters of the ITAs are measured and corrected for magnification, at the desired level from the first to the seventh costal cartilages. This is quite reliable because the ITAs lie virtually in one plane in their entire intrathoracic course. Beyond the seventh costal cartilage, the ITAs enter the rectus sheath and do not lie in the same radiographic plane. Therefore, beyond this point, the measurements become unreliable. Only posteroanterior radiographic views should be used for estimation of the arterial diameter.

ANATOMY OF THE ITAs

Textbooks of anatomy have given an inadequate description of the anatomy of the ITAs, probably because the surgical importance of these vessels was not realized until recent interest in myocardial revascularization occurred. The anatomy described below is based on the author's experience with bilateral selective opacification of the native ITAs in over 300 subjects.

ITA Origin

In 98% of the subjects, the ITAs arise from the anteroinferior aspect of the first part of the subclavian artery as it arches over the apex of the lung. Within the first part, the origin is variable. For angiographers, the most important radiographic landmark is the medial end of the clavicle in the posteroanterior view. The ITA orifice is usually slightly lateral and above it. Due to the asymmetry of the aortic arch branches, the distance from the origin of the left subclavian artery to the ITA orifice is smaller than the distance from the origin of the right innominate artery to the ITA orifice (Fig. 3–3A,B). In elderly and hypertensive patients with a high aortic arch, the innominate artery may become extremely tortuous (Fig. 3–3B), making the right ITA catheterization using a femoral approach difficult or impossible. In patients with a low aortic arch, tortuosity is minimal (Fig. 3–3A) and catheterization using a femoral approach is not difficult unless atherosclerosis is present.

Some anatomical variants should be mentioned here. Origin of the ITA from the third part of the subclavian artery, as the vessel crosses the first rib, occurs 2% of the time on the right side and 1% of the time on the left side (Fig. 3–4A,B). This is of surgical importance. Such a vessel takes a very divergent course above the first costal cartilage, and the vessel may become injured during proximal surgical dissection (Fig. 3–5).

In 4% of the cases, the suprascapular artery shares a common origin with the ITA (Fig. 3–6). This artery is usually a branch of the thyrocervical trunk. In 1% of cases, the ITA and the entire thyrocervical trunk come off the subclavian artery as a single trunk (Fig. 3–7). I do not believe that these anatomical variants have any bearing on the surgical result (Fig. 3–8).

Course and Termination

From their origin, the ITAs incline downward and medially behind the medial end of the clavicle, entering the thorax behind the first costal cartilage and descending approximately 1.5 to 2 cm from the lateral sternal border to bifurcate in 50% of cases within the limits of the sixth intercostal space. In the other 50%, the artery bifurcates either above or below this point. This is usually no higher than the fifth and no lower than the seventh costal cartilage. The terminal branches are the musculophrenic and superior epigastric arteries (Fig. 3–9). The musculophrenic artery courses laterally and downward, supplying the diaphragm and contributing intercostal branches to the lowest intercostal spaces. The superior epigastric artery usually passes vertically downward into the rectus sheath to anastomose with the branches of the inferior epigastric artery.

In about 10% of cases, the superior epigastric artery does not descend through or behind the rectus abdominis muscle but swings sharply laterally, somewhat parallel to the musculophrenic branch (Fig. 3–9, middle panel). In these cases, a large branch is given off, descending vertically, in the lateral part of the rectus abdominis, and anastomosing below with the inferior eipgastric artery.[2] This anatomical variation is important to the surgeon attempting very distal dissection of this vessel.

Another important anatomical variant is the high bifurcation at the third or fourth costal cartilage level (Fig. 3–10), occurring in 2% of patients bilaterally. This is of surgical importance. Limited dissection in the midthoracic region may result in one branch being grafted and the other left intact.[3] This results in diversion of graft flow.

The two terminal branches are rarely equal in caliber. If surgical dissection is performed beyond the bifurcation, the larger branch should be used for

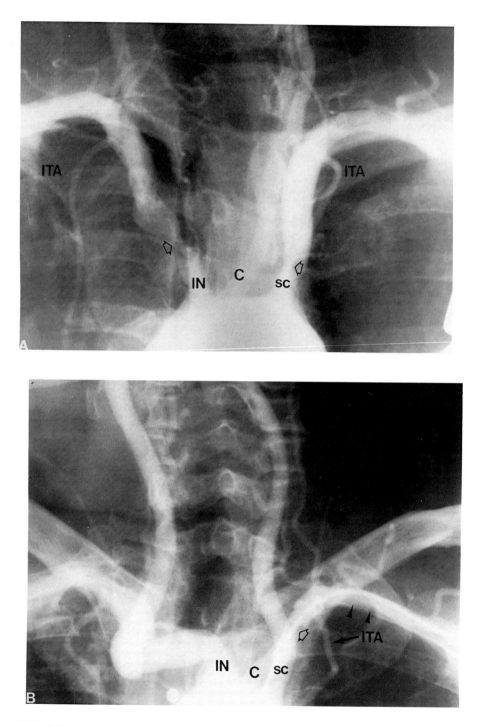

FIGURE 3–3 Aortic arch studies. **A:** Low aortic arch. Severe bilateral brachiocephalic disease is seen (arrows). Both ITAs were normal. IN = innominate artery; SC = left subclavian artery; C = carotid artery. **B:** High aortic arch. Atherosclerosis of the left subclavian artery (SC) is seen proximal (arrow) and distal (arrowheads) to the left ITA. C = carotid artery. (From Singh RN: Atherosclerosis and the internal mammary arteries. *Cardiovasc Intervent Radiol* 6:72–77, 1983.)

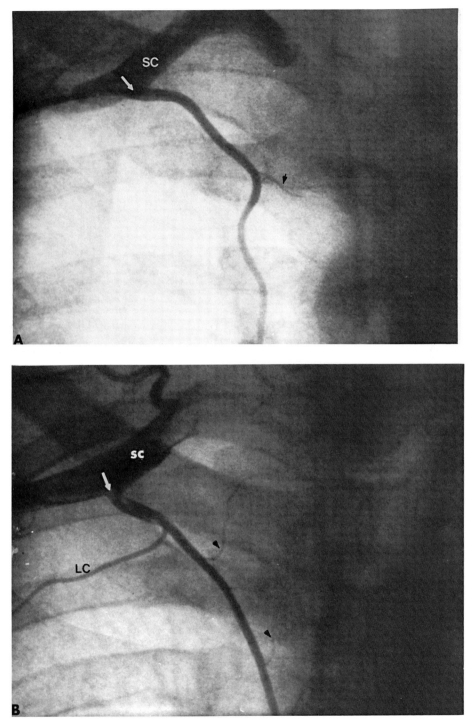

FIGURE 3–4 A,B: Anomalous origin (arrow) of the right ITA from the third part of the subclavian artery (SC). Thymic branches (arrowheads) and the lateral costal branch (LC) are seen.

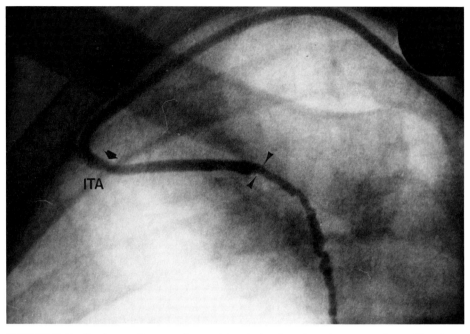

FIGURE 3–5 Postoperative angiographic study showing the anomalous distal origin (arrow) of the ITA. The beaded appearance beyond the arrowheads is caused by thermal injury. (Courtesy of T.C. Sharma, M.D.)

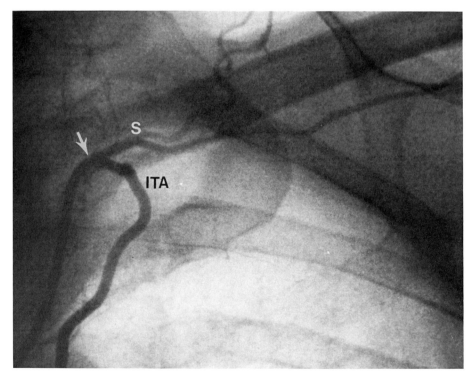

FIGURE 3–6 Common origin (arrow) of the left ITA with the suprascapular branch (S). (From Singh RN: Radiographic anatomy of the internal mammary arteries. *Cathet and Cardiovas Diagn:* 373–386, 1981

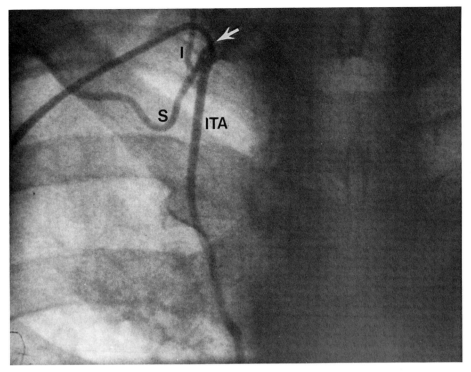

FIGURE 3–7 Common origin (arrow) of the right ITA with the thyrocervical trunk. S = supracapsular branch; I = inferior thyroid artery. (From Singh RN: Radiographic anatomy of the internal mammary artery. *Cathet and Cardiovasc Diagn* 7:373–386, 1981.)

grafting. If both branches are of adequate caliber (Fig. 3–9, right panel), a natural Y graft is feasible for two coronary arteries lying close together. Rarely, no terminal branching is seen, and the distal ITA directly enters the rectus sheath (Fig. 3–11).

Branches of the ITA

Very small ITA branches are poorly visualized arteriographically. This is due to rapid dissipation of injection pressure because of very free anastomosis of ITA branches in the intercostal spaces as well as terminally in the rectus sheath. These small branches have been well outlined by Arnold[2] by means of postmortem angiography in specially prepared cadaver specimens. The major branches are described below.

Lateral Costal Branch

This inconstant branch was known to the early anatomists and is termed the "accessory mammary artery" in the old anatomical literature.[4] It has been erroneously described in recent surgical literature as the first intercostal branch. The vessel is not confined to the intercostal space. It arises at or above

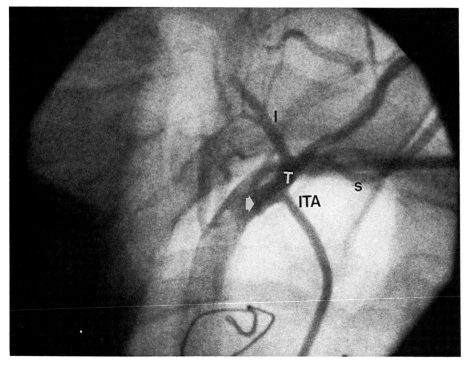

FIGURE 3-8 Postoperative angiographic study showing the common origin (arrow) of the left ITA and the thyrocervical trunk (T). Note the good caliber of the ITA graft, indicating absence of the steal phenomenon.

the first costal cartilage and courses subpleurally, laterally, and downward into the lateral chest wall (Fig. 3–12A). The artery is sizable in 10% of cases, usually bilaterally, and its size depends upon its length in the lateral chest wall, where it can travel several intercostal spaces, giving intercostal branches.[5] It may be as large as the ITA. Such a large artery, if not divided during mobilization of the ITA pedicle, may cause tenting of the ITA graft and diversion of flow to the lateral chest wall.[6] Dissection of this vessel from the chest wall for use as an additional in situ coronary graft is possible and has been described.[7]

A vestigial, small-caliber lateral costal branch which ends anteriorly is found in another 10% of cases, either unilaterally or bilaterally (Fig. 3–12B). Such a rudimentary lateral costal branch is not capable of large runoff and is not of surgical importance.

Mediastinal Branches

Small branches pass backward, supplying mediastinal pleura and areolar tissue. These may arise from the sternal branches or directly from the ITA. Those arising opposite the manubrial segment of the sternum supply the thymus and the thymic fat (Fig. 3–4A,B). In about 25% of cases, a large branch arises from the back of the ITA below the manubriosternal joint and sweeps posteri-

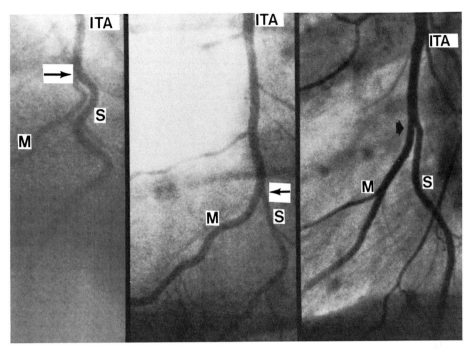

FIGURE 3-9 Distal segment of the right ITA in three patients showing bifurcation into the superior epigastric (S) and musculophrenic (M) arteries. The left panel shows a large superior epigastric and a small musculophrenic branch. The middle panel shows a small superior epigastric and a large musculophrenic branch. The right panel shows a high division and equally large superior epigastric and musculophrenic branches. (From Singh RN, Taylor PC: Use of the right mammary artery for coronary bypass. *Vascular Surgery* 21:301–304, 1987. Published by Westminster Publications.)

orly at an acute angle to supply the anterior pericardium and adjacent mediastinal pleura. This may be designated the "major anterior pericardial branch" (Fig. 3–12A).

Anatomy textbooks describe a constant branch that accompanies the phrenic nerve between the pleura and the pericardium. It has been termed the "pericardiophrenic branch." Arteriographically, it is frequently seen, but not 100% of the time. Often, multiple long pericardial branches are seen coming off the upper part of the ITA (Fig. 3–13).

The major anterior pericardial branch and the long pericardial branches have potential for developing collaterals to the pulmonary circulation via the subpleural mediastinal plexus.[5] This may occur after ITA grafting and may cause a reduction of flow to the grafted coronary artery.[6]

Sternal Branches

The sternal branches arise opposite each intercostal space and pass medially toward the sternum. They bifurcate near its lateral margin into branches

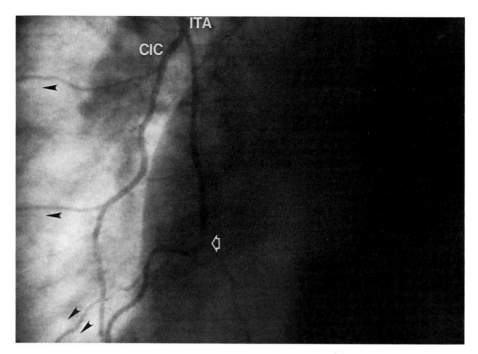

FIGURE 3-10 Distal segment of the right ITA showing high bifurcation at the third costal cartilage level into a lateral (CIC) and a medial branch (open arrow). (From Singh RN, Taylor PC: Use of the right mammary artery for coronary bypass. *Vascular Surgery* 212:301–304, 1987.)

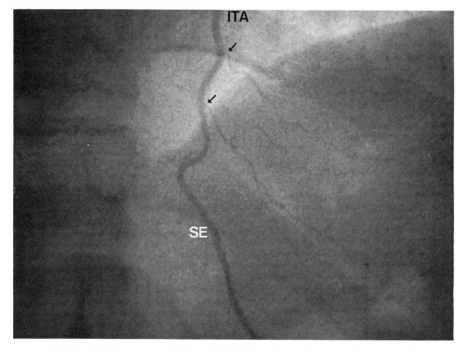

FIGURE 3-11 Distal segment of the left ITA showing absence of terminal bifurcation and direct continuation as the superior epigastric artery (SE). Lower intercostal branches are shown by arrows.

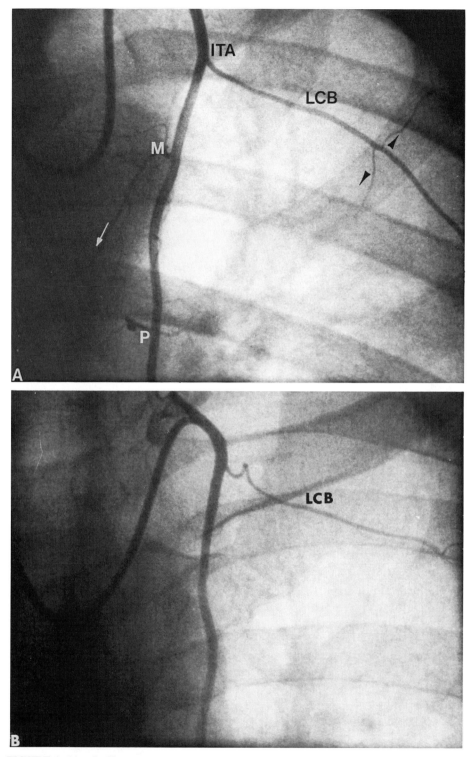

FIGURE 3–12 A: Upper part of the left ITA showing a large lateral costal branch (LCB), a major anterior pericardial branch (M), and a perforating branch (P). **B:** Upper part of the left ITA showing a small lateral costal branch (LCB). (From Singh RN: Radiographic anatomy of the internal mammary arteries. *Cathet and Cardiovasc Diagn* 7:373–386, 1981.)

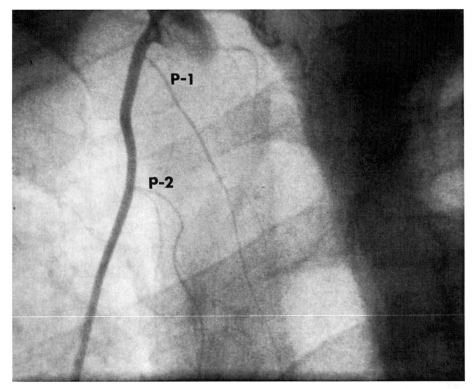

FIGURE 3-13 Left anterior oblique view of the upper part of the right ITA showing long pericardial branches near the origin (P-1) and at the level of the first costal cartilage (P-2). (From Singh RN: Radiographic anatomy of the internal mammary arteries. *Cathet and Cardiovasc Diagn* 7:373–386, 1981.)

which pass into the anterior and posterior periostea. These small branches are often not visualized arteriographically.

Intercostal Branches
In the upper three or four intercostal spaces, small branches of the ITA pass directly laterally along the upper and lower borders of the costal cartilage. The lower intercostal branches are often larger (Figs. 3–14, 3–15), and it is increasingly common for a single trunk to be given off opposite the costal cartilage, pass downward and outward, and then divide into two branches running along the upper and lower borders of the costal cartilage.

Perforating Branches
A perforating branch is given off at almost all of the first five intercostal spaces. However, not all of these are visualized arteriographically. There is usually one large perforating branch on each side at the upper end of the sternum. These branches penetrate the internus, the external membrane, and the pectoralis major and may bend laterally to supply the integument. The

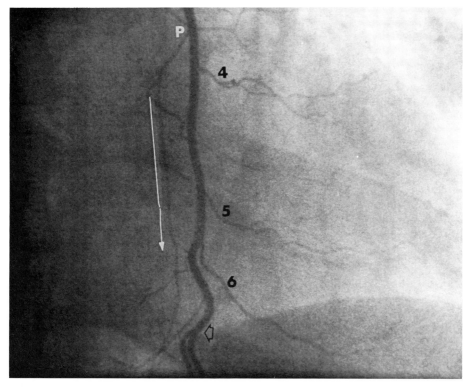

FIGURE 3–14   Distal part of the left ITA showing small branches to the fourth, fifth, and sixth intercostal spaces (4, 5, 6) and the terminal division (open arrow). A long pericardial branch (P) arises from the fourth space. (From Singh RN: Radiographic anatomy of the internal mammary arteries. *Cathet and Cardiovasc Diagn* 7:373–386, 1981.)

perforating branches are directed medially at their origin and bend laterally to cross the ITA and course toward the lateral chest wall (Fig. 3–16). In this respect, these branches are arteriographically different from the intercostal branches. In some interspaces, intercostal and perforating branches arise from a common stem. In patients with unusually large lower intercostal and/or large perforating branches, the caliber of the distal ITA may become very small at the point of bifurcation (Fig. 3–16).

Size of the Internal Thoracic Arteries

Arteriography is the most reliable method of estimating the size of the ITA.[5] ITA caliber correlates poorly with age, sex, or body size.[1] In 98% of subjects, the diameter exceeds 1.5 mm at the level of the fourth costal cartilage (Fig. 3–17). This is why the left ITA is nearly always suitable for grafting the anterolateral coronary arteries. At this level, the diameters of the right and left ITAs are nearly always identical. For the ITA graft to reach the posterior

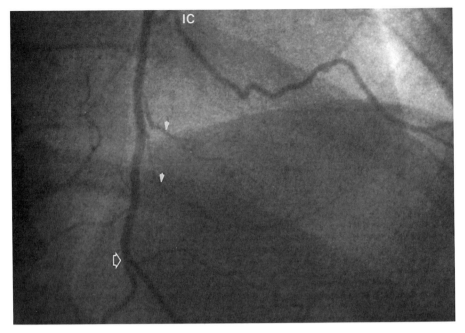

FIGURE 3–15 Distal part of the left ITA showing an unusually large intercostal branch (IC) at the third costal cartilage level. Arrowheads show small lower intercostal branches. The terminal bifurcation is shown by the open arrow.

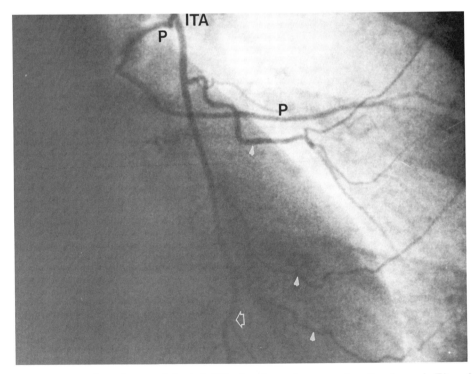

FIGURE 3–16 Distal part of the left ITA showing a large perforating branch (P) and lower intercostal branches (arrowheads). The terminal bifurcation is shown by the open arrow. Note the minuscule terminal branches.

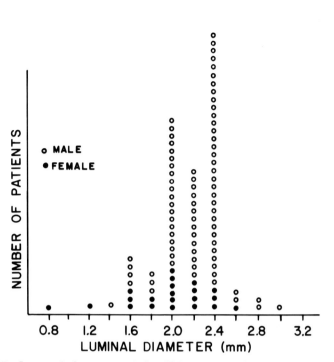

INTERNAL MAMMARY ARTERY IN 100 PATIENTS

FIGURE 3–17 Luminal diameter of the ITAs measured at the level of the fourth costal cartilage in 100 patients. (From Singh RN: Radiographic anatomy of the internal mammary arteries. *Cathet and Cardiovasc Diagn* 7:373–386, 1981.)

coronary circulation, the ITA caliber needs to be adequate at or beyond the bifurcation. At this level, there is no bilateral symmetry in caliber. Arteriographically, the estimated ITA diameter at the site of anastomosis should be 1.5 mm or greater.[8] One of the two terminal branches of the ITA meets this criterion in over 75% of cases. Figures 3–18 and 3–19 illustrate a very large and a very small ITA, respectively.

Atherosclerosis

The incidence of atherosclerosis in the ITAs is approximately 2%.[9] The common site of atherosclerosis is the distal segment around the terminal bifurcation (Fig. 3–20). This usually does not interfere with grafting unless a very long pedicle is required. There is less than a 1% incidence of significant atherosclerosis at the origin of the ITA. Such a vessel cannot be used as an in situ graft. Atherosclerosis of the subclavian arteries (Fig. 3–3A,B) occurs in 4% of patients with coronary artery disease and is a contraindication for in situ ITA grafting if the lesion is proximal to the ITA origin.

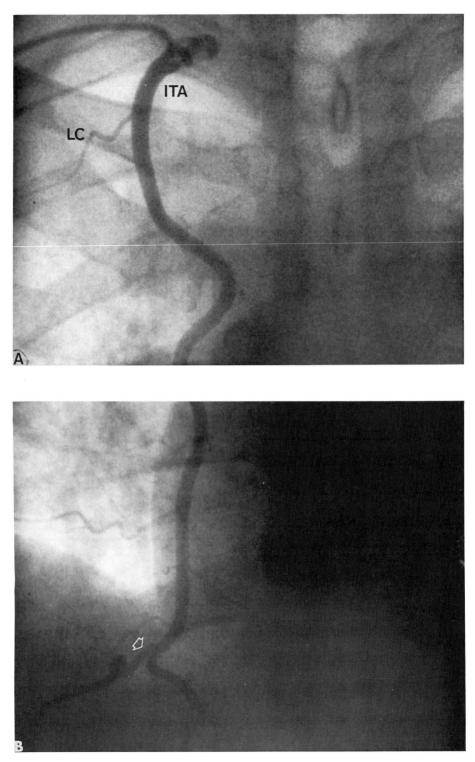

FIGURE 3–18 Proximal (**A**) and distal (**B**) parts of a very-large-caliber right ITA. A small lateral costal branch (LC) is also seen. The terminal bifurcation is shown by the open arrow.

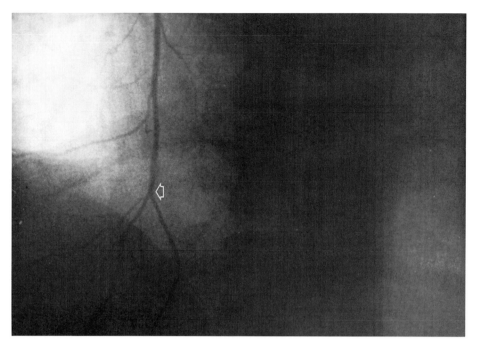

FIGURE 3–19 Distal part of a very-small-caliber right ITA. The terminal bifurcation is shown by the open arrow. Note the minuscule terminal branches.

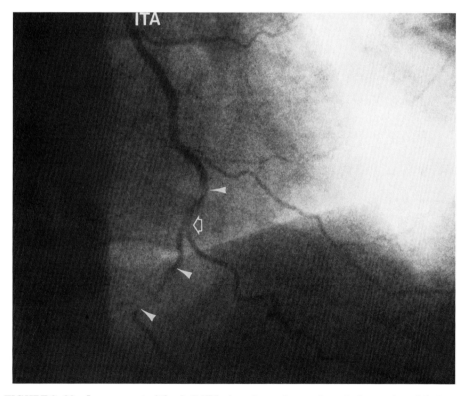

FIGURE 3–20 Lower part of the left ITA showing atherosclerosis (arrowheads) above and below the bifurcation (open arrow). (From Singh RN: Atherosclerosis and the internal mammary arteries. *Cardiovasc Intervent Radiol* 6:72–77, 1983.)

REFERENCES

1. Singh RN: Internal mammary arteriography: A new catheter technique by right brachial approach. *Cathet Cadiovasc Diagn* 6:439–449, 1980.
2. Arnold M: The surgical anatomy of sternal blood supply. *J Thorac Cardiovasc Surg* 64:596–610, 1972.
3. Schmid C, Heublein B, Reichelt S, et al: Steal phenomenon caused by a parallel branch of the internal mammary artery. *Ann Thorac Surg* 50:463–464, 1990.
4. Kropp B: The lateral costal branch of the internal mammary artery. *J Thorac Surg* 21:421–425, 1951.
5. Singh RN: Radiographic anatomy of the internal mammary arteries. *Cathet Cardiovasc Diagn* 7:373–386, 1981.
6. Singh RN, Sosa JA: Internal mammary artery–coronary artery anastomosis: Influence of the side branches on surgical result. *J Thorac Cardiovasc Surg* 82:909–914, 1981.
7. Hartman AR, Mawulawde KI, Derban JP, et al: Myocardial revascularization with the lateral costal artery. *Ann Thorac Surg* 49:816–818, 1990.
8. Singh RN, Taylor PC: Use of the right mammary artery for coronary bypass. *Vascular Surg* 21:301–304, 1987.
9. Singh RN: Atherosclerosis and the internal mammary arteries. *Cardiovasc Intervent Radiol* 6:72–77, 1983.

CHAPTER 4

Postoperative Evaluation of the ITA Grafts

J.A. SOSA

BACKGROUND

The ITA has gained great popularity as a coronary artery bypass conduit since its first utilization.[1] The relative prevalence of arteriosclerotic heart disease and its complications has made coronary artery bypass surgery an important modality, if not the cornerstone, of its treatment. More than two decades ago, Favaloro reported successful aortacoronary bypass surgery using autologous saphenous vein grafts.[2] Also during the last two decades, it became evident that saphenous vein grafts have a significant incidence of late occlusions.[3] The ITA began to be used as an alternative coronary bypass conduit in 1968.[4] Initially, this alternative modality quickened the interest of those working in the field. Analysis of the experience with postoperative opacification of the ITA revealed an increase in its use between 1970 and 1975. However, for somewhat ill-defined reasons, this interest dwindled from 1975 to 1985. Reports began to appear in the literature in 1980[5] and 1983[6] documenting the enhanced long-term patency of the ITA as a coronary artery bypass conduit; as a result, a resurgence in its use has been noted. From that time to the present (Fig. 4–1), an increasing number of centers have advocated and expanded the use of bilateral, sequential, and free ITA bypass grafts in order to improve the long-term results.[7] The surgical technique involved in the use of the ITA as a conduit in coronary artery bypass surgery requires scrupulous attention to minute detail.[7] For this reason, in order to ascertain and document the adequacy of the surgical results, periodic randomly chosen postoperative angiographic studies should be performed.

My experience in opacifying ITAs dates back to 1960, when I was a cardiology fellow at the Cleveland Clinic's Cardiac Catheterization Laboratory under the direction of Dr. F. Mason Sones, Jr. That early experience came while learning to opacify, consistently and safely, the left ITA in patients who had

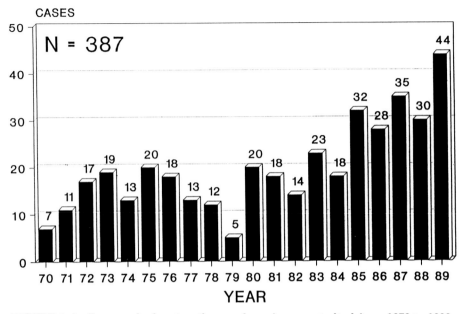

FIGURE 4–1 Bar graph showing the number of cases studied from 1970 to 1989.

undergone left ITA implants (Vineberg operation) to either the anterior or lateral wall of the left ventricular chamber. From 1960 to 1970, a straight No. 7F or No 8F Cordis* aortic DSA catheter was used. The tip of these catheters was shaped like a "hook" (Fig. 4–2) with the aid of a sterile "straightened paper clip" which was introduced into the end hole of the catheter and then shaped into various-sized hooks. Once the catheters were shaped, they were immersed in sterile boiling normal saline, thus achieving the required permanent contour. With these catheters, a virtually 100% success rate was achieved when using an arterial cutdown in the ipsilateral arm.

In 1970, the Cordis Corporation began manufacturing an ITA catheter (Fig. 4–3) which could be used via a cutdown or via the percutaneous femoral approach. From 1970 to 1980, this catheter was used ipsilaterally. In 1980, Dr. R.N. Singh, then at Montefiore Hospital in Pittsburgh, in cooperation with the Cordis Corporation, developed a special catheter with acute primary and secondary 80° curves for cannulation of the ITA from the contralateral arm (Fig. 4–4). This catheter allows cannulation of the contralateral ITA in 87% of cases and cannulation of the ipsilateral ITA in 100%.

In selectively opacifying the ITAs, I have used the cutdown retrograde brachial approach exclusively. Difficulties with the percutaneous femoral method have been reported[8] and are well known. These complications include structural damage, as well as failure to achieve close to 100% selective yield. To achieve a high yield and to prevent structural damage, more cumbersome methods (variations of the percutaneous femoral technique) have been pro-

---

*Cordis Corporation, P.O. Box 025100, Miami, FL 33102-5700.

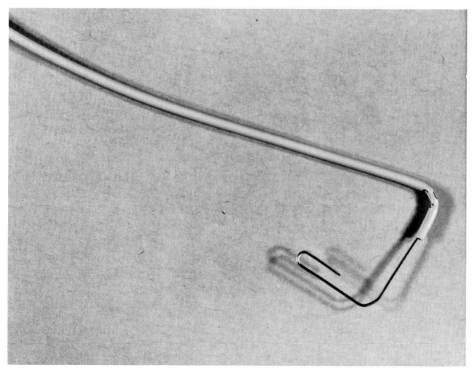

FIGURE 4–2 Aortic DSA catheter (Cordis) shaped with a sterile paper clip.

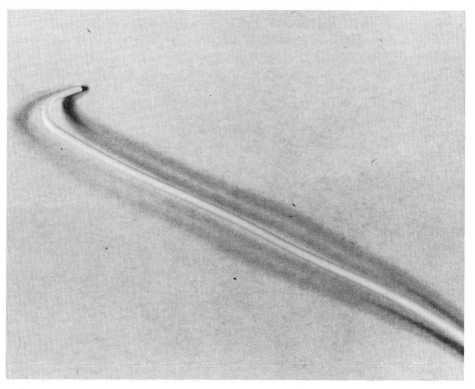

FIGURE 4–3 Standard ITA catheter (Cordis) usable via brachial cutdown or via percutaneous femoral puncture.

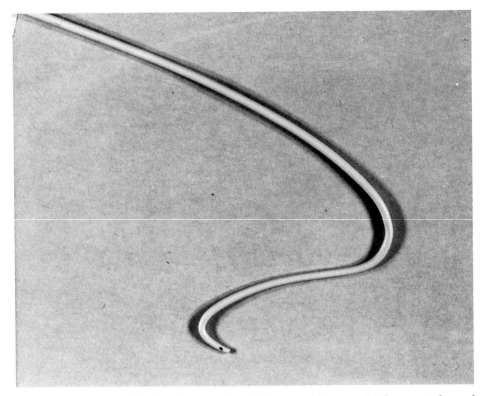

FIGURE 4-4 Special ITA catheter (Cordis) designed to opacify the contralateral artery from the ipsilateral arm.

posed. These have merit, and they do aid those limited to such an approach. The cutdown retrograde brachial approach using the ipsilateral or contralateral arm has proven extremely safe, with 100% yield, and thus is recommended. Nonselective methods of ITA angiography have been described[8] and presently are undergoing clinical trials. The basic concept uses a balloon-tipped catheter (Fig. 4–5) with a proximal port for dye injection. This catheter can be placed in the right or left subclavian artery just beyond the takeoff of the ITA. The balloon is inflated with CO_2 until the distal port pressure waveform confirms obstruction of blood flow into the axillary artery. Power injections of contrast material are carried out through the proximal port, thus achieving opacification of the ITA. The disadvantage of these methods is that large volumes of contrast material need to be injected, which is of concern when the neighboring vertebral artery may be the recipient of some, if not a large portion, of the injection.

A somewhat more ambitious concept is being tested at our laboratory. This consists of using a balloon-tipped catheter with a proximal port which also has a second balloon proximal to the side port (Fig. 4–6). Upon inflation of both balloons, the origin of the given ITA is isolated, limiting the injection to the corresponding ITA.

Semiselective intra-arterial digital subtraction arteriography has been

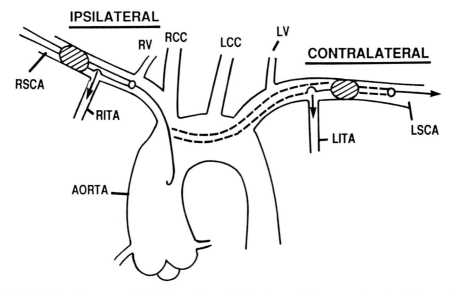

FIGURE 4–5 Diagram of a balloon-tipped catheter used for nonselective ITA opacification.

mentioned as an acceptable nonselective method to opacify ITAs in the postoperative period.[9] R wave gated digital subtraction arteriography relies on low-dose, slow injections of dilute contrast material into the origin of the innominate or corresponding subclavian artery. The proponents of this method initially expressed doubts about its reliability and its value as a clinical tool, and although subsequent reports have endorsed its usefulness, the procedure has significant drawbacks.

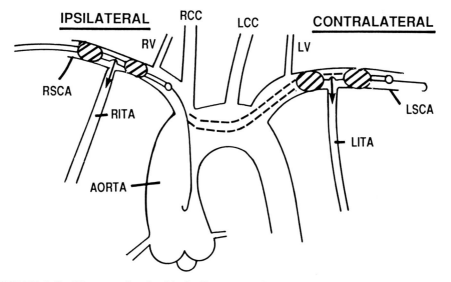

FIGURE 4–6 Diagam of a double balloon-tipped catheter used for nonselective ITA opacification.

TABLE 4-1 Summary of Patient Population Profile

Total Number of Patients		387	Total Number of ITA's	491
Sex	Male	317	LITA (Single)	261
	Female	70	RITA (Single)	22
Age	Range	16–87	LITA & RITA	104
	Average	63		
			Average Time Postoperatively	
Study Methods			Until Angiogram	
Right arm only		219	LITA	58 Months
Left arm or combined		168	RITA	13 Months

On principle, it goes contrary to established wisdom in advocating a nonselective technique over a selective one. The experience with the coronary arteries does not substantiate that claim. Enough detail is never obtained with nonselective techniques. In addition, the amount of contrast material used, although dilute, is considerably larger than it would be if a selective modality was used, and therefore neighboring arterial systems are exposed to it. This is particularly important in reference to the corresponding vertebral artery.

Another significant obstacle is the cost of the radiological equipment necessary to carry it out. Those concerned with cost containment in health care consider digital systems as valuable ancillaries, but not essential.

Finally, the ipsilateral or contralateral arm approach, as described here, has proven safe and rich in necessary detail. Nonselective techniques prove useful in cases of anomalous origin of the ITAs, but it is doubtful that they will replace the presently acceptable selective methods.

EXPERIENCE

From 1960 to 1970, the cutdown retrograde ipsilateral arm technique was perfected during work with ITA implant patients. The definitive report of a coronary artery bypass with the ITA was published in 1968. In a fortuitous manner, and because of my experience, I had the opportunity at that time to begin opacifying the left ITA when directly anastomosed end-to-side to either the anterior descending or circumflex artery. Over the last two decades, I have had the opportunity to study 387 symptomatic patients postoperatively. All the studies were performed using the cutdown retrograde selective ipsilateral or contralateral brachial artery technique employing standard or specially designed ITA catheters.* The patient population profile is summarized in Table 4-1. Of these patients, 317 (82%) were male and 70 (18%) were female. The ages ranged from 16 to 87 years, with an average age of 63. Of the studies, 261 (67%) concerned the single left ITA and 22 (5%) concerned the right ITA. In addition, 104 (27%) were studies of both ITAs, for a total of 491 single separate selective studies of an ITA in a grafted position to the diseased coronary arterial tree. The average time for a postoperative angiographic study

*See Figs. 4-3 and 4-4.

of the single left ITA was 58 months, while for the single right ITA it was 13 months. A total of 219 studies (57%) were completed using the right arm only; in the remaining 168 (43%), either the left arm or both arms were used. Early complications consisted of two left subclavian artery dissections (distal to the origin of the ITA), both while using the catheter shown in Fig. 4–3, and one brief transient cerebral ischemic attack. There were no deaths or other late complications. All the angiographic studies included at least two oblique views of each artery, with the x-ray beam at the corresponding right angles. The early experience was gained using undiluted 76% ditriozoate, but it was soon learned that in approximately 90% of the patients, the selective injections of 5 to 10 cc of this undiluted contrast agent produced a brief but very painful sensation in the anterior chest (commonly in the distribution of the corresponding ITA). For that reason, by 1971, selective ITA injections were made using various degrees of diluted (with 5% glucose and water) 76% ditriozoate to a minimum of 50%. This was done until the advent of nonionic or low-osmolarity contrast agents around 1983–1985, when it was learned that these new agents did minimize, if not completely abolish, the painful experience referred to above. From that point on, routine practice has been to use the new agents in severely symptomatic patients and the standard 76% ditriozoate in various degrees of dilution in all others. Of the new agents, ioxaglate* was found to be most tolerable.[9]

The frequency of postoperative ITA angiographic studies has increased over the last two decades. This increment reflects the more frequent utilization of the ITA as a coronary bypass conduit by cardiac surgeons. In 1978, only 8% of North American cardiac surgeons reported using at least one ITA in myocardial revascularization operations. This figure rose to 47% in 1986. With the increase in the number of these operations, there has been a proportionate increment in the number of postoperative studies necessary to elucidate the possible causes of recurrent anginal symptoms. During 1970–1979, the yearly number of cases peaked in 1975, when 20 were studied. The number of cases studied decreased to 5 in 1979. From that point on, the number of cases has steadily increased, peaking in 1989, whens 44 cases were studied (Fig. 4–1).

RESULTS

Table 4–2 summarizes the results of the cineangiographic studies done on 365 ITAs. Of the total, only 104 (29%) (Fig. 4–7) were judged to meet the criteria for adequacy. Adequacy is defined as a left ITA graft gently coursing from the left subclavian artery to the corresponding diseased native coronary artery, displaying initial integrity, no more than 10% loss of caliber from its origin to the distal anastomosis, and no excessive tortuosity (redundancy) or kinking. In addition, prominent side branches such as the lateral costal and/or pericardiophrenic arteries should not be identifiable. These angiographic characteristics indicate that the surgical technique employed avoided the inadequacies listed in Table 4–2.

---

*Hexabrix, Mallinckrodt Medical, Inc., 675 McDonnell Boulevard, St. Louis, MO 63402.

TABLE 4–2 Summary of LITA Results

Adequate	104
Distal narrowing >50% narrowing of grafted native vessel	75
Side–to–side narrowing >50%	34
Prominent lateral costal artery	35
Redundancy and tortuosity	26
Exagerated angulation	16
Pericardial phrenic branches	15
End–to–side narrowing >50%	9
Torsion	9
Kinked	7
Thermal injury	3
Competitive flow	2
Total occlusion	1
Isolated luminal narrowing	1
Diffuse loss of caliber (Free-standing graft)	16
Progression of native disease	10
Partial obstruction	2
	Total = 365

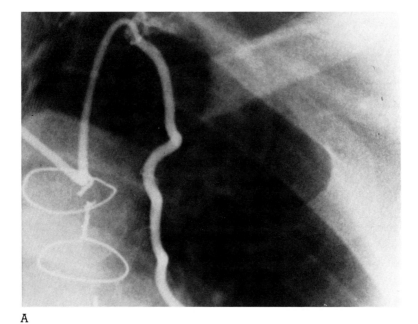

A

FIGURE 4–7 A–C: LITA displaying the characteristics of adequacy.

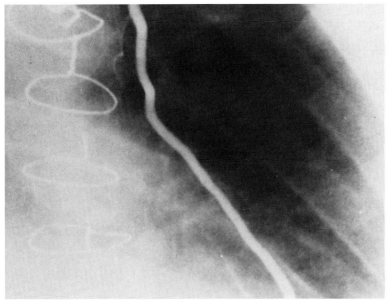

B

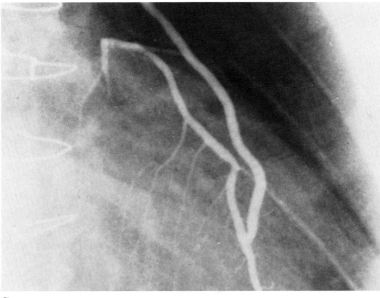

C

FIGURE 4-7 Continued

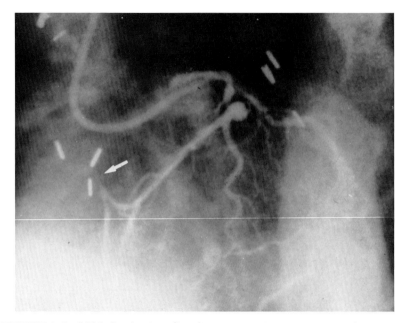

FIGURE 4–8   LITA displaying distal anastomotic narrowing with tension.

The small percentage of adequate ITA grafts seems to indicate that although the left ITA is being used with greater frequency and by more cardiac surgeons, proper surgical technique is not widely practiced. It is essential that surgeons presently using the technique review the details of it, and that those without experience but wishing to begin using it make the effort necessary to carry it out according to established guidelines.

Seventy-five left ITAs (LITA) (Fig. 4–8) displayed 50% or more distal anastomotic narrowing with 50% or more luminal narrowing of the grafted vessel near the anastomosis. Fifty-seven of these cases displayed tension suggesting inadequate graft length.

Thirty-four (9%) LITAs (Fig. 4–9) displayed inadequate side-to-side anastomosis with narrowing of 50% or more at the anastomotic site, with corresponding flow restriction to the native grafted vessel.

Thirty-five (10%) LITAs (Fig. 4–10) displayed a prominent lateral costal branch with a caliber of 50% or more of that of the LITA itself. The prominence acquired by this branch has suggested to many observers the possibility of siphoning blood flow away from the diseased grafted coronary vessel and thus representing the possibility of diversion of flow. Detailed analysis of these angiographic studies do show the lateral costal branch's growth in caliber, as well as the briskness of its blood flow. It is important to note that all these patients were symptomatic (i.e., had anginal syndrome), and in seven cases, thallium stress testing showed reversible ischemia in the distribution of the LITA in question (personal experience). In at least one patient (Fig. 4–10), embolization of the lateral costal branch was considered as a therapeutic alter-

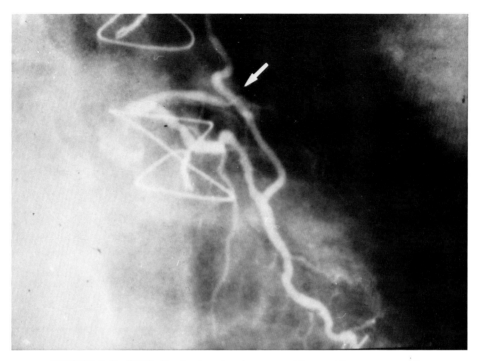

FIGURE 4-9 LITA displaying inadequate side-to-side anastomosis.

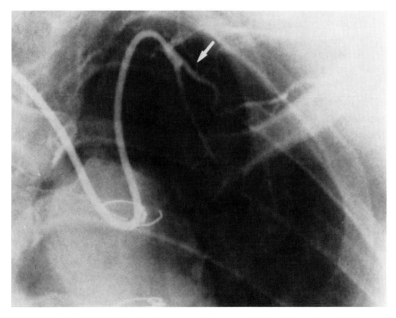

FIGURE 4-10 LITA displaying prominence of the lateral costal branch.

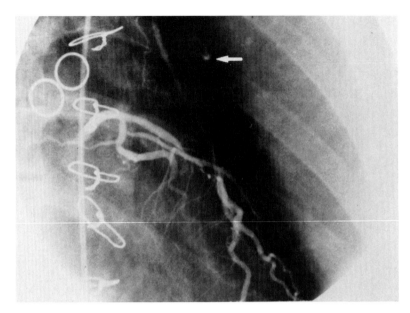

FIGURE 4–11 LITA displaying prominent pericardiophrenic branches.

native but was never performed. At the time of this writing, the patient is on medical treatment.

Fifteen (4%) LITAs (Fig. 4–11) displayed prominent pericardiophrenic branches suggesting the possibility of diversion of flow. In two of these patients, this flow diversion was noted to exist between the pericardiophrenic branches and the lung parenchyma. One patient underwent reoperation because of recurrence of symptoms judged to be due to progression of disease in a previously normal right coronary artery and to the existence of the fistulous flow. Reoperation confirmed the presence of the flow diversion to lung parenchyma (personal communication with Dr. G. Green). This finding is akin to the problem presented by the prominent lateral costal artery referred to above. The cardiac surgeon should sever all LITA branches from the terminal portion to the subclavian origin.

Thirty-three (9%) LITAs (Fig. 4–12) displayed significant redundancy and marked tortuosity, indicating that the graft was not tailored adequately. Seven (1.9%) of these LITAs (Fig. 4–13) displayed sharply defined, abrupt luminal discontinuations resembling a "kink." In redundant grafts, attempts to advance coronary angioplasty guide wires through these kinks commonly prove difficult, requiring stiffer wires and deeper intromission of the guiding catheter. Conceivably, these angiographic abnormalities could constitute flow impedance leading to an inadequate supply of oxygen to the myocardium.

Sixteen (4%) LITAs (Fig. 4–14) displayed exaggerated angulation at the site of side-to-side anastomosis, also with distal loss of caliber of the segment between the side-to-side and distal anastomoses. This represents a difficulty with the side-to-side anastomotic technique that seems key but that not all surgeons agree upon.

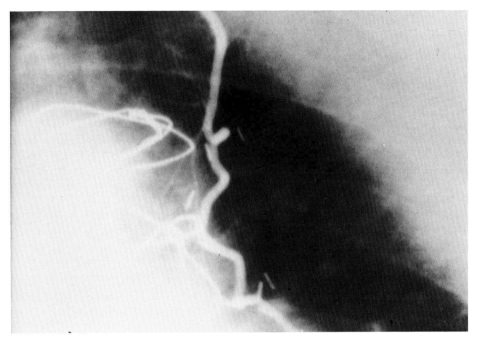

FIGURE 4–12 LITA displaying redundancy.

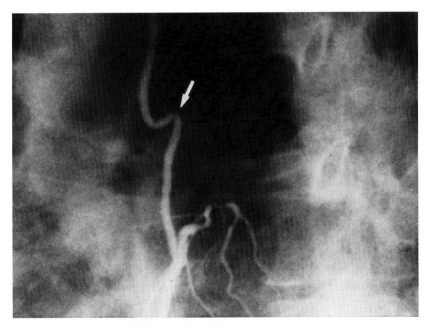

FIGURE 4–13 LITA displaying kinks.

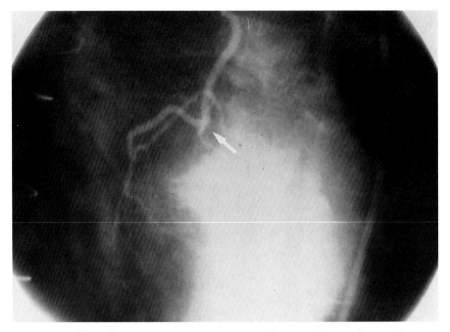

FIGURE 4–14 LITA displaying exaggerated angulation of the side-to-side anastomosis, with loss of caliber in the distal segment to the end-to-side anastomosis.

Nine (2.5%) LITAs (Fig. 4–15) displayed inadequacy of the end-to-side anastomosis (luminal narrowing of at least 50%) when the LITA was part of a more proximal side-to-side anastomosis.

Nine (2.5%) LITAs (Fig. 4–16) displayed a well-defined loss of luminal caliber (most of it in the middle), showing luminal "grooving." In shape, the grooving is reminiscent of a folded umbrella and is likely to show at the point where the twisting took place. This angiographic abnormality is referred to as "torsion." It was confirmed as such when two patients were reoperated on because of the reappearance of symptoms.

Three (0.82%) LITAs (Fig. 4–17) displayed diffuse and full-length intimal irregularities with appreciable loss of luminal caliber (intimal "feathering"). These changes are attributable to thermal injury resulting from an inappropriately high-energy setting of the cautery used in the preparation of the LITA pedicle. These postoperative angiographic findings occurred in three patients operated on during a specific time period which coincided with the use of a new cautery. This fact was confirmed by analysis of the operative records.

One (0.27%) LITA (Fig. 4–18) appeared to be totally occluded, showing as a blind stump. This was the only totally occluded LITA in the entire series, which shows its rarity.

Two (0.27%) LITAs (Fig. 4–19) displayed a significant loss of caliber (50% or more of the contralateral vessel) in the course of the graft, particularly in the distal half proximal to and including the distal anastomosis. The native grafted vessel is visualized filling well in a retrograde fashion, suggesting "competitive flow," which in turn signifies overestimation of the severity of the

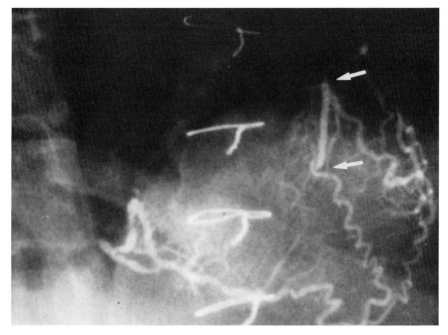

FIGURE 4–15 LITA displaying narrowing of the end-to-side anastomosis when a side-to-side anastomosis also exists.

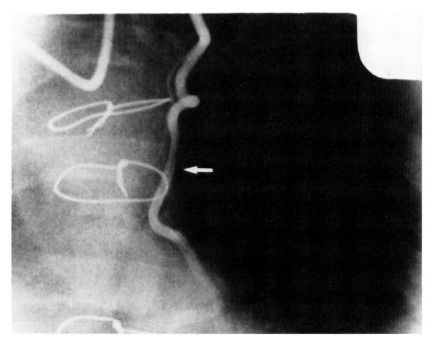

FIGURE 4–16 LITA displaying the grooving site of torsion.

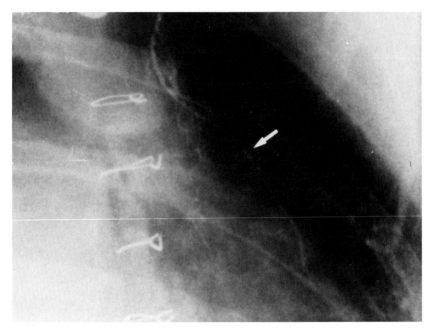

FIGURE 4–17 LITA displaying feathering and loss of lumen caliber representing thermal injury.

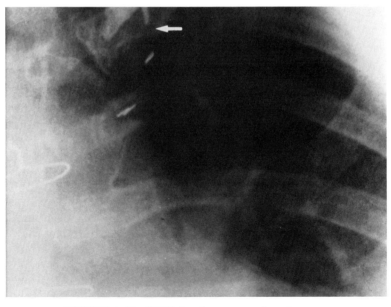

FIGURE 4–18 LITA displaying total occlusion.

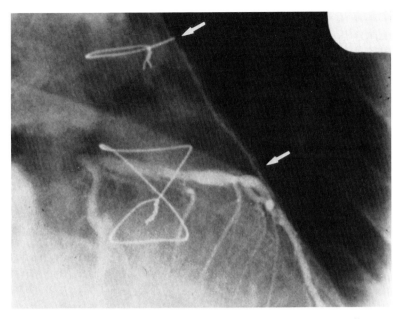

FIGURE 4-19 LITA displaying changes due to competitive flow.

preoperative lesion. This overestimation has been confirmed by corresponding antegrade angiographic studies of the vessels in question. The LITA is a very sensitive live conduit which adapts to the different physiological needs of myocardial blood flow. Competitive flow leads to its diminution in caliber.

One (0.27%) LITA (Fig. 4–20) displayed discrete, well-defined luminal narrowing in the very proximal segment of the graft. The etiology of this abnormality is unclear, although it was observed only once. It did not respond to intravascular or sublingual nitroglycerin.

Sixteen (4%) LITAs (Fig. 4–21) were used as free-standing grafts from the proximal aorta to the branches of the left coronary artery system. All of these grafts displayed significant reduction (50% or more) of their caliber (Fig. 4–21) from the proximal to the distal anastomosis. Flow appeared less than optimal.

In 10 (3%) of the LITAs (Fig. 4–22) studied, progression of disease in the native circulation was found. It was somewhat surprising how infrequently this occurred. All of these cases involved postoperative angiographic studies performed at least 10 years after surgery.

Two (0.5%) LITAs (Fig. 4–23) were partially obstructed when the neighboring left subclavian artery was dissected during selective cannulation attempts. This constitutes procedural morbidity, which can be minimized by using the right catheter (see Fig. 4–4) and by keeping the tip of the catheter away from the inferior surface of the corresponding subclavian artery.

Postoperative angiographic studies of right ITAs (RITAs) show a somewhat different profile. It is apparent that some of the technical difficulties were avoided due to the experience gained when utilizing the LITAs. However, tension has been a common problem with the RITA pedicle grafts, probably

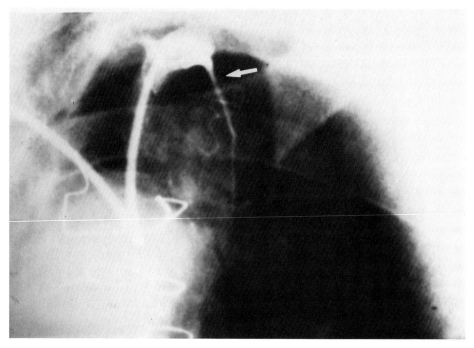

FIGURE 4–20 LITA displaying proximal well-defined narrowing.

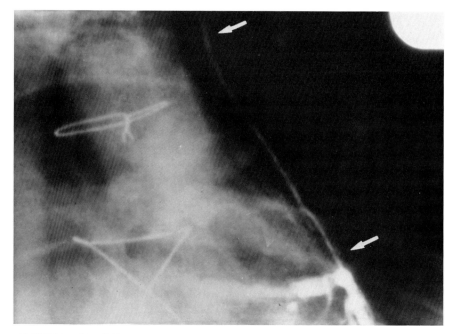

FIGURE 4–21 LITA displaying changes noted when placed as a free graft.

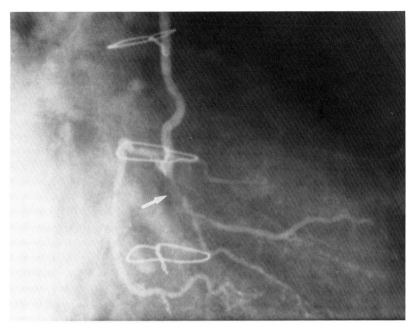

FIGURE 4–22 LITA anastomosed to native vessels displaying significant progression of disease.

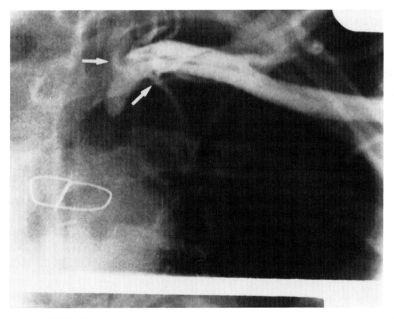

FIGURE 4–23 LITA displaying partial obstruction and dissection of the neighboring subclavian artery.

TABLE 4–3 Summary of RITA Results

Adequate	47
Tension–inadequate length	63
Distal narrowing >50%	12
Thermal injury	2
Torsion	1
Total occlusion	1
Total =	126

due to their inadequate length when not used as free grafts. Table 4–3 summarizes the results of the angiographic studies done on 126 RITAs.

Sixty-three (50%) RITAs (Fig. 4–24) displayed tension or pulling, indicating inadequate length. This is manifested by uniform caliber loss with a very straight course.

Forty-seven (37%) RITAs (Fig. 4–25) met the criteria of adequacy as described for the LITAs (see above). It is interesting that a larger percentage of RITAs were found to meet the criteria of adequacy. This can be explained by the fact that RITAs began to be used well during the time when technical experience with the LITA had been defined. Many of the technical surgical difficulties has been ironed out by the time the RITAs became common in coronary bypass surgery.

Twelve (9.5%) RITAs (Fig. 4–26) displayed inadequacy of the distal anastomosis (luminal narrowing of 50% or more). This abnormality is clearly akin to the same abnormality visualized in the postoperative LITA studies.

Two (1.6%) RITAs (Fig. 4–27) showed diffuse intimal irregularities of the

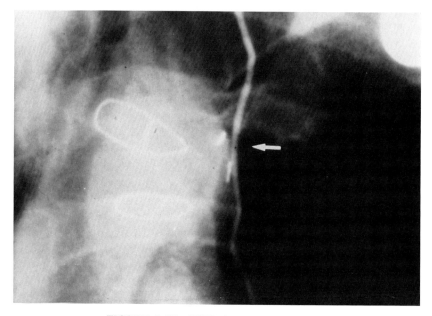

FIGURE 4–24 RITA displaying tension.

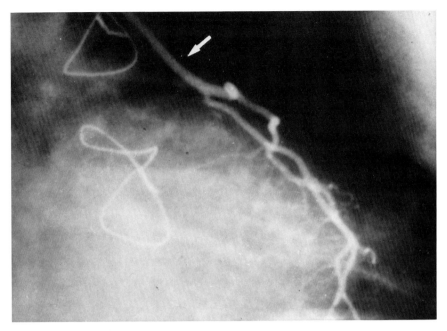

FIGURE 4-25 RITA displaying findings described as adequate.

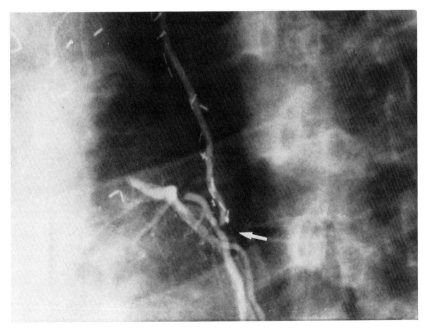

FIGURE 4-26 RITA displaying narrowing of the distal anastomosis.

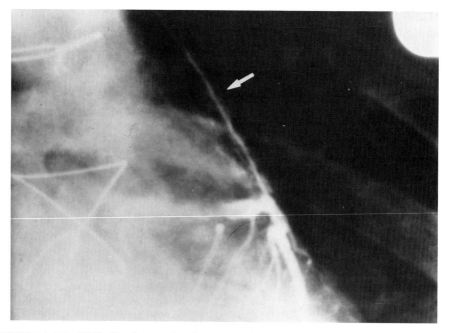

FIGURE 4–27 RITA displaying feathering and loss of lumen caliber representing thermal injury.

entire length of the graft, with appreciable loss of lumen caliber (intimal feathering) attributable to thermal injury. These two cases were the result of an inappropriate high-energy setting of the cautery used in the preparation of the RITA pedicle. The patients were operated on sequentially with the LITA patients noted to have similar findings, as mentioned above.

One (0.8%) RITA (Fig. 4–28) appeared as a stump, indicating total obstruction of the graft.

Two (0.8%) RITAs (Fig. 4–29) displayed well-defined loss of luminal caliber with intimal grooving indicating torsion.

The data base used for this analysis represents the work of nine different cardiac surgeons from five different geographical regions of the United States.

CONCLUSIONS

Certain valid conclusions can be drawn from this analysis.

Unquestionably, both ITAs are being used with greater frequency as conduits in myocardial revascularization operations, as well as by more cardiac surgeons.

As documented by postoperative angiographic studies, it is clear that the patency rate of the ITAs, when interposed as myocardial revascularization conduits, is greatly superior to that of autologous vein grafts.

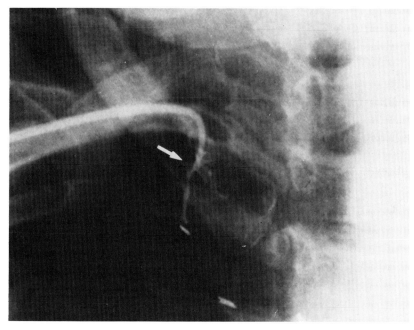

FIGURE 4–28 RITA displaying total obstruction.

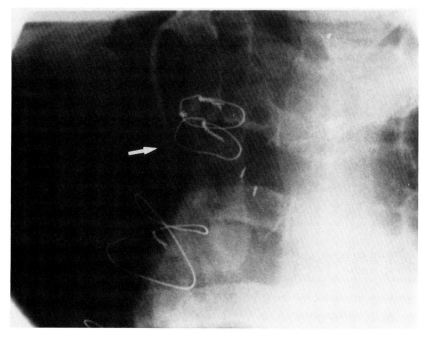

FIGURE 4–29 RITA displaying grooving or torsion.

Anastomotic surgical techniques are far from perfect and there is no general consensus as to how best to achieve it.

Contralateral and ipsilateral brachial retrograde ITA angiography has proven safe and acceptable. Attention to detail is mandatory, and adherence to proper procedural technique assures relative patient safety and precise results.

REFERENCES

1. Kolesov VI: Mammary artery-coronary artery anastomosis as treatment for angina pectoris. *J Thorac Cardiovasc Surg* 54:535, 1967.
2. Favaloro RG: Saphenous vein autograft replacement of severe segmental coronary occlusion. *Ann Thorac Surg* 5:334–339, 1968.
3. Campeau L, Enjalbert M, L'Esperance J, et al: Comparison of late changes (closure and atherosclerosis at 10 years) in internal mammary artery and saphenous vein coronary grafts. *Circulation* 68:114, 1983.
4. Green GE, Stertzer SH, Reppert EH: Coronary arterial bypass grafts. *Ann Thorac Surg* 5:443–450, 1968.
5. Jones JW, Ochsner JL, Mills NL, et al: Clinical comparison between patients with saphenous vein and internal mammary artery as a coronary graft. *J Thorac Cardiovasc Surg* 80:334–341, 1980.
6. Singh RN, Sosa JA, Green GE: Long-term fate of the internal mammary artery and saphenous vein grafts. *J Thorac Cardiovasc Surg* 86:359–363, 1983.
7. Green GE, Sosa JA, Cameron A: Prospective study of feasibility of routine use of multiple internal mammary anastomoses. *J Thorac Cardiovasc Surg* 30:643–647, 1989.
8. Kuntz RE, Baim DS: Internal mammary angiography: A review of technical issues and newer methods. *Cathet Cardioivasc Diagn* 20:10–16, 1990.
9. Rankin VS, Newman GE, Bashore TH, et al: Clinical and angiographic assessment of complex IMA bypass grafting. *J Thorac Cardiovasc Surg* 92:832–846, 1968.
10. Davies RF, LeMay M, Beanlands DS, et al: Comparison of ioxaglate with ditriozoate in angiography of the internal mammary artery. *Cathet Cardiovasc Diagn* 15:11–14, 1988.

CHAPTER 5

Clinical Results of Internal Thoracic Artery Bypass Surgery

AIRLIE A. C. CAMERON

With abundant evidence of the internal thoracic artery's (ITA's) resistance to atherosclerosis, whether the artery is examined in situ[1] or as a coronary artery bypass graft,[2] it could be anticipated that clinical results of patients with ITA bypasses would be superior to that of patients dependent on vein grafts alone. However, for many reasons, this evidence was slow in being reported. These reasons include selection of vein grafts by the majority of surgeons in the early years of bypass surgery, the learning curve associated with use of the ITA, the late appearance of vein graft failure, the lack of use of ITA grafts in large multicenter clinical trials, and bias in the choice of conduit in certain patient groups.

Although the ITA was first used as a direct coronary artery bypass graft in this country in 1968, most surgeons used the technically easier saphenous vein bypass procedure almost exclusively; thus, large groups of patients were not available for clinical follow-up. Since ITA–coronary artery anastomoses are more technically demanding than the vein graft procedure, the early patency rates and thus the early clinical results tend to reflect either the learning curve or the expertise and experience of the individual surgeon rather than the properties of the grafts themselves. Although the patency rates of ITA grafts generally exceed those of vein grafts in the immediate postoperative period, it is only with increasing years that the rapid attrition of vein grafts due to accelerated atherosclerosis becomes apparent[3] and the wide disparity in patency rates becomes evident. The ITA graft is less prone to late atherosclerosis, a major determinant of the clinical result, but this attribute is not apparent immediately after surgery.

The major multi-institutional clinical trials in the 1970s, namely, the VA Cooperative Study, the European Cooperative Study Group, and the Coronary

Artery Surgery Study (CASS), did not include the ITA as a randomizing feature, and only in CASS were ITA grafts reported as performed at all. There was only one small, randomized trial[4] comparing the clinical results of ITA and saphenous vein grafts. It is now unlikely that there will ever be a larger such trial, as nonrandomized observational studies have documented superior clinical results with the ITA grafts.

Comparison of ITA and vein graft recipients is made more difficult by the tendency of surgeons to show bias not only in deciding which patients receive ITA grafts but also in deciding to which coronary artery the ITA graft is anastomosed. In some centers, surgeons avoid use of the ITA in women, in older age groups, and in those with impaired ventricular function, recent infarctions, or emergency operations. In addition, the ITA is usually placed to the left anterior descending coronary artery (LAD), which generally supplies the largest area of myocardium and the area most commonly responsible for fatal myocardial infarctions.[5] Most follow-up studies have evaluated patients with single (usually left) pedicled ITA grafts with single coronary anastomoses. Studies of bilateral versus single, right versus left, free versus pedicled, and sequential versus single anastomoses are still controversial or the results undecided.

RANDOMIZED TRIALS

The single reported prospective randomized trial comparing vein grafts with ITA grafts began in 1975[4] and involved 80 patients. The patients, all with single-vessel disease, received a graft to the LAD and were randomly assigned to the ITA group (39 patients) or the vein graft group (41 patients). Their baseline characteristics were remarkably similar, although the two groups were not stratified for the usual risk factors, including ventricular function. By 10 years, with an excellent overall follow-up of 97.5% in the study group, there was a significantly better survival in the ITA group compared to vein graft group (92.3% and 82.1%, respectively), as well as greater freedom from all cardiac events. Although this study is small and the two groups were not stratified for known predictors of mortality, the study is unique because it is the only one in which the choice of conduit was randomly assigned.

SURVIVAL STUDIES WITH A SINGLE ITA GRAFT

Results of observational studies in large clinical populations became available in the 1980s. Reports of 10-year follow-up studies comparing ITA and saphenous vein graft procedures appeared in 1984[2] and 1986,[6] 12-year follow-up studies in 1984,[7] 15-year follow-up studies in 1986,[8] and a 9-year follow-up study in 1989.[9] One study has now been extended to 19 years.[10] All of these reports (Table 5–1) were single-institution studies, with groups of patients ranging in size from 278[2] to 5,931.[6] In addition, a multi-institutional study with 6,977 patients from 15 institutions reported a 7-year follow-up study in

TABLE 5-1 Comparison of survival rates in patients with an ITA graft with or without additional vein grafts and in patients with vein grafts alone

| Author | Years of Follow-up | Internal thoracic artery | | Veins | | p value |
		No. of Patients	Survival (%)	No. of Patients	Survival (%)	
Acinapura et al.[9]	9	2,100	90	1,753	78	<.01
Grondin et al.[2]	10	40	84.3	238	70	
Loop et al.[6]	10	2,306	86.6	3,625	75.9	<.0001
Okies et al.[7]	10	259	82	139	69	<.002
Cameron et al.[8]	14	532	72	216	57	<.01
Cameron and Green[10]	19	490	55	214	35	<.01

1988.[11] These studies were primarily with single pedicled grafts, although one study[8] included bilateral grafts in 38 patients. None of the studies were randomized. Although the clinical features varied between the vein graft and ITA groups, multivariate analysis in three of the studies[6,8,11] identified the ITA as an independent predictive factor in survival. The reductions in the risk of dying associated with an ITA graft noted in these three studies were remarkably similar: 0.62,[6] 0.65,[8] and 0.64.[11] The survival rates in the five studies in Table 5-1 cannot be compared because some studies[6] did not include operative mortality in the overall survival rate and some excluded patients with emergency surgery,[6,9] evolving myocardial infarction,[6,9] or significant left main coronary artery stenosis.[6] Patients undergoing reoperations or additional surgery, such as valvular procedures or aneurysm resection, were excluded in all studies. Some studies[6,7,9] included only patients receiving an ITA or vein graft to the LAD, with or without additional grafts. In spite of these differences in patient subgroups, all studies concluded that the presence of an ITA was a significant contributor to survival.

The Cleveland Clinic study,[6] involving 5,931 patients, showed that the 10-year survival with an ITA graft was significantly better than with vein grafts alone in single-vessel (93.4% vs. 88%, $p = .05$) (Fig. 5-1), double-vessel (90% vs. 79.5%, $p < .0001$) (Fig. 5-2), and triple-vessel disease (82.6% vs. 71%, $p < .0001$ (Fig. 5-3). The ITA graft was placed to the LAD in all patients. Improved survival with an ITA graft was noted in men as well as women and in those with normal to mildly impaired ventricular function as well as those with moderate to severe impairment. The CASS analysis[11] demonstrated that by 7 years the presence of an ITA graft was associated with improved survival (Table 5-2), not only in men and women, in those with normal and near-normal or impaired ventricular function, but also in patients with and without left main coronary artery stenosis, as well as in older and younger patients. The CASS analysis included 15 clinical centers, with use of the ITA graft ranging from 0 to 66.2% of each center's operations. The survival rates were better in patients with an ITA graft, whether operated on at a center commonly or infrequently using the ITA bypass procedure. Thus, the CASS and Cleveland Clinic experiences conclusively demonstrate that the bias in selec-

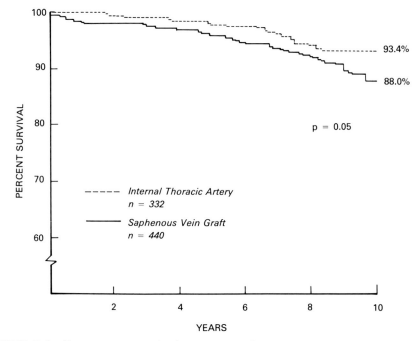

FIGURE 5–1 Ten-year survival of patients with one-vessel (anterior descending artery) disease who had either an isolated ITA graft or a vein graft. The survival difference was statistically significant by univariate analysis; however, when preoperative multivariate characteristics were entered, significance was lost. (From Loop FD, et al: Influence of the internal-mammary-artery graft on 10-year survival and other cardiac events. *N Engl J Med* 314:1–6, 1986.)

TABLE 5–2 Cumulative survival rates at 7 years in patients with an ITA graft with or without associated vein grafts compared with patients with vein grafts only from the CASS Registry

	Internal thoracic artery		Vein graft		
	No. of patients	Survival (%)	No. of patients	Survival (%)	*p* value
Left ventricular score <10	711	93	4,032	89	.004
Left ventricular score ≥10	221	84	1,776	71	.004
Left main coronary artery stenosis <50%	858	92	5,215	84	<.0001
Left main coronary artery stenosis ≥50%	91	90	801	79	.051
Men	798	91	4,988	84	<.0001
Women	152	90	1,037	79	.005
Age ≤65 years	881	92	5,405	85	<.0001
Age >65 years	69	88	620	69	.01

Source: Cameron A, et al: Clinical implications of internal mammary artery bypass grafts: The Coronary Artery Surgery Study experience. *Circulation* 77:815–819, 1988.

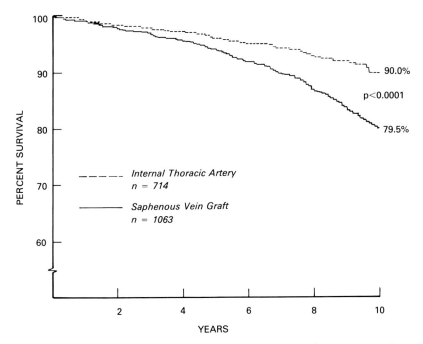

FIGURE 5-2 Ten-year survival of patients with two-vessel disease, including those with lesions of the proximal anterior descending artery. The difference in survival between the patients who received ITA grafts and those who received saphenous vein grafts was significant by both univariate and multivariate analysis. (From Loop FD, et al: Influence of the internal-mammary-artery graft on 10-year survival and other cardiac events. *N Engl J Med* 314:1–6, 1986.)

tion of the ITA as a conduit in terms of sex and ventricular function, and in the CASS experience for age and left main coronary artery stenosis as well, was not warranted. These studies have extended the use of the ITA to these subgroups of patients. In addition, the CASS observation that the benefit of the ITA graft was seen at centers infrequently utilizing this conduit should encourage surgeons who have not used this graft to begin employing it.

RECURRENCE OF ANGINA

Angina pectoris, a subjective symptom, is difficult to quantify. Thus, the incidence of recurrent angina following bypass surgery varies considerably among reports. However, meaningful observations can be made from comparisons between patients with and without ITA grafts at a single institution or among several institutions when definitions are carefully standardized. The reasons for recurrence of angina include early graft failure, usually attributed to technical difficulties at operation; late graft failure; and progression of disease in the coronary arteries. Many centers have documented progressive graft failure in saphenous veins but not in ITA grafts, as well as evidence[12] of more rapid progression in native coronary arteries with less than 50% lesions when by-

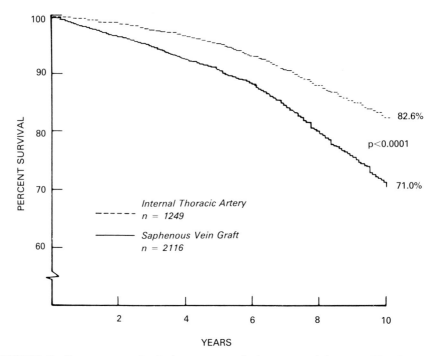

FIGURE 5-3 Ten-year survival of patients with three-vessel disease. The ITA group contained those who had one ITA graft and one or more saphenous vein grafts. The saphenous vein graft group had vein grafts only. The difference between the two groups was significant by both univariate and multivariate analysis. (From Loop FD, et al: Influence of the internal-mammary-artery graft on 10-year survival and other cardiac events. *N Engl J Med* 314:1–6, 1986.)

passed with a saphenous vein graft compared with an ITA graft. Thus a beneficial effect of the ITA graft on recurrence of angina would be expected, and this indeed was documented.[8,9,11]

Acinapura et al.,[9] in a 9-year study, compared 2,100 patients with ITA grafts to 1,753 patients with vein grafts only. They found a cumulative probability of recurrent angina by 9 years in 30.6% of patients in the vein graft group compared with 18% of patients in the ITA graft group ($p < .01$). These authors also noted that in patients with recurrent angina, those with ITA grafts had less need for reoperation than those with vein grafts. Presumably, the angina was less severe or the demonstrated coronary artery disease was less life-threatening in the ITA group than in the vein graft group. Loop et al.[6] noted that at 10 years patients with vein grafts had 1.2 times the risk of postoperative angina ($p = .004$) of patients with ITA grafts to the LAD.

The authors of a 15-year study[8] noted significantly less recurrent angina ($p < .01$) in the first year in patients with an ITA graft; however, thereafter, the annual recurrence rate (3.2% and 3%, respectively) did not differ between those receiving an ITA graft and those receiving vein grafts only (Fig. 5–4). By 15 years approximately 70% of those still alive in either group had experienced angina of any severity. It was noted that the cumulative survival rates in patients with postoperative angina and an ITA graft were better ($p < .01$)

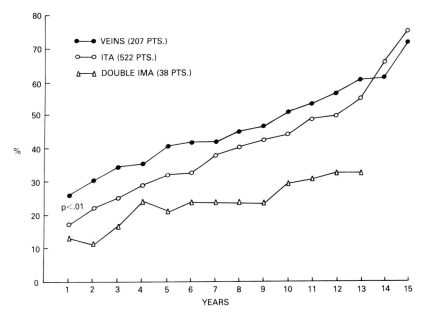

FIGURE 5-4 Annual recurrence rate of angina pectoris in patients receiving vein grafts only and in patients with a single or double ITA graft, with or without additional vein grafts. (From Cameron A, et al: Bypass surgery with the internal-mammary-artery graft: 15-year follow-up. *Circulation* 74:III-30–III-36, 1986.)

than in those with angina and vein grafts alone. Presumably, in both groups, progression of disease and failure of associated vein grafts played major roles in the recurrence of angina.

LATE MYOCARDIAL INFARCTIONS AND REOPERATIONS

Other clinical manifestations of recurrent coronary atherosclerosis, such as late myocardial infarction, need for reoperation, and need for hospitalization for cardiac reasons, have been studied. At the Cleveland Clinic,[6] it was noted that by 10 years there was a 1.41 times risk of late myocardial infarction ($p < .001$), 1.25 times risk of hospitalization for cardiac events ($p < .0001$), and 1.27 times risk of all late cardiac events ($p < .0001$) in patients with vein grafts only, compared with patients receiving ITA grafts to the LAD. ITA grafts conferred no advantage in terms of reducing cardiac arrhythmias, suggesting that arrhythmias are dependent on a mechanism different from that responsible for the return of angina, late myocardial infarction, the need for reoperation, or death, all of which are reduced by the presence of an ITA graft to the LAD.

Okies et al.[7] noted that at 12 years there was an improved event-free survival in patients who had received left ITA grafts. Events included severe angina, congestive heart failure, myocardial infarction, and death. This was true even in the group with a single graft to the LAD ($p < .04$). In a 15-year

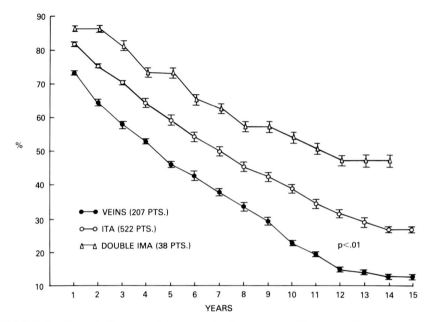

FIGURE 5–5 Cumulative event-free survival rates over 15 years of patients receiving vein grafts alone, or single or double ITA grafts with or without additional vein grafts. (From Cameron A, et al: Bypass surgery with the internal-mammary-artery graft: 15-year follow-up. *Circulation* 74:III-30–III-36, 1986.)

study,[8] patients with ITA grafts had fewer myocardial infarctions ($p < .02$), fewer reoperations ($p < .001$), and better cumulative event-free survival ($p < .01$) (Fig. 5–5). The mortality rates associated with these late infarctions, while not significantly different, showed better protection with ITA grafts than with vein grafts alone (29.6% with vein grafts alone compared with 16.6% with ITA grafts). There was no information on the location of these late infarctions, but it is possible that the improved mortality rates in the ITA graft group can be attributed to sparing of the anterior wall due to a patent ITA graft to the LAD. When this study was extended to 19 years,[10] 54% of the vein-graft-only group compared to 38% of the single-ITA group had had a late myocardial infarction. In the vein-graft-only group, 28% required reoperations compared to only 13% of the single-ITA group after 19 years of follow-up. Mortality rates associated with these reoperations were similar: 7.5% in both groups, with or without a prior ITA graft.

BILATERAL ITA GRAFTS

With evidence of better clinical results with a single ITA graft, it could be anticipated that still further improvement in clinical results would be seen in patients with bilateral ITA grafts. An early study[13] in 1982 reporting on 76 patients with bilateral ITA grafts demonstrated excellent survival (90.2%) at 9 years. The grafts included 33 free ITA grafts and 43 pedicled grafts. There were no comparison groups in this study or in a 12-year study reported in

1985[14] involving 227 patients. These patients had an 83% actuarial survival at 10 years, with 69% being asymptomatic at that time, as well as a low incidence of late myocardial infarction and need for reoperation.

When comparisons between bilateral and single ITA grafts were made, a disparity in patency rates between right and left ITA grafts was noted in some reports. In a study of 814 patients with ITA grafts,[15] repeat angiography over a 10-year period showed significantly better patency rates for left ITA compared with right ITA grafts. Indeed, the patency rates of right ITA grafts were no different from those of saphenous vein grafts. The technical difficulties with right ITA grafts and the resultant reduced patency rates would clearly affect the clinical results. In 1989 a 15-year study[16] of 6,181 consecutive patients showed no increased benefit with multiple ITA grafts, although there was a significant benefit in terms of survival with an ITA graft compared with a vein graft. The patient groups were not stratified for known predictors of survival other than age, and no angiographic data were available. These data would be required before it could be concluded that bilateral ITA grafts conferred no additional benefit in terms of survival and recurrent clinical manifestations of coronary artery disease compared with that obtained from a single ITA graft.

In 1990 Fiore and colleagues,[17] in a 15-year study of 200 patients, demonstrated a significant additional benefit of bilateral compared to single ITA grafts. The grafts were all pedicled grafts without sequential grafting. The patients in the two groups of 100 each were similar for known predictors of survival. Of great importance, the patency rates at 13 years were similar in the right and left ITAs. There were significantly improved clinical results in the bilateral ITA group compared with the single ITA group in terms of better survival ($p = .01$), fewer myocardial infarctions ($p < .025$), less recurrent angina ($p < .025$), and fewer total ischemic events ($p < .01$) during the 15-year follow-up period. With angiographic evidence of similar patency rates in both ITA grafts, this clinical follow-up evaluated not the operative technical problems associated with performing a right ITA graft but rather the functional effectiveness of bilateral vs. single ITA grafts over the long term. The conclusion from other studies that bilateral ITA grafts do not confer additional clinical benefit probably reflect the increased technical problems of utilizing the right ITA as a coronary bypass graft.

Another 15-year report[8] included 38 patients with bilateral ITA grafts in a study comparing 207 patients with vein grafts only to 522 patients receiving ITA grafts with or without additional vein grafts. The patients with bilateral ITA grafts had the best cumulative survival rates (Fig. 5–6) and the least recurrence of angina (Fig. 5–4) and needed no reoperations during the 15-year follow-up. No angiographic data were reported in this study, but with such improved results with bilateral over single ITA grafts, it can be assumed that the patency rates were similar in the right and left ITAs.

FREE ITA GRAFTS

When free (aortocoronary) ITA grafts were first proposed, there was concern that the relative immunity from atherosclerosis demonstrated in the ITA pedi-

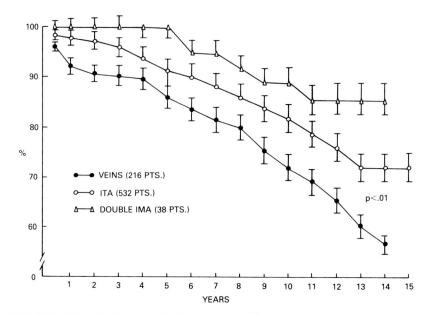

FIGURE 5-6 Cumulative survival rates over 15 years of patients receiving vein grafts alone, or single or double ITA grafts with or without additional vein grafts. (From Cameron A, et al: Bypass surgery with the internal-mammary-artery graft: 15-year follow-up. *Circulation* 74:III-30–III-36, 1986.)

cled graft would be adversely affected by impairment of the lymphatic drainage and vasovasorum of the ITA when used as a free graft. However, early reports[18] demonstrated an excellent patency rate of 89.8% in the 49 patients with free ITA grafts restudied at 10.7 months. Of the 29 patients receiving a free ITA as their only graft, only 5 failed to improve in the early postoperative period. In a later study[19] from the same institution, 156 patients with free ITA grafts, as well as those with associated pedicled ITA and saphenous vein grafts, were evaluated. The 10-year survival rate was 73.3%, and of the free ITA grafts restudied, 84% were patent. In addition, there was no evidence of atherosclerosis in the free ITA grafts. Although there may be technical difficulties with anastomoses of the ITA to the aorta, particularly to an atherosclerotic aorta, the late patency rate of the ITA as a free graft appears to be as good as that of the pedicled ITA graft. Thus, the clinical result of patients with free grafts would be expected to parallel that of patients with pedicled ITA grafts.

SEQUENTIAL GRAFTS

Sequential grafting increases the number of coronary vessels approachable with ITA grafts and may result in complete revascularization utilizing ITA grafts only.[20,21] There have been no clinical studies comparing the results of patients with sequential grafts and those with single anastomotic sites. In a series of 41 patients with sequential ITA grafts supplying complete revascularization to the left ventricle,[20] of the 38 patients followed for an average of 1 year, only one reported angina during this time and was demonstrated to have graft stenosis. Another study with 100 patients[22] with an average 3.2 ITA grafts as well as associated vein grafts reported no angina during early follow-up. The clinical follow-up of patients with sequential ITA grafts will depend on the patency of the graft, as adequate flow reserves to both the proximal and distal anastomotic regions has been demonstrated in sequential ITA grafts.[23]

CONCLUSIONS

From many observational studies and a single randomized study, the use of an ITA graft with or without additional vein grafts has consistently yielded clinical results superior to those obtained with the use of vein grafts alone. These improved results include better long-term survival, less early return of angina, fewer late myocardial infarctions, and less need for reoperation. These findings have been confirmed at many centers for single pedicled ITA grafts and appear to be true as well for free grafts, bilateral grafts, and sequential grafts.

The improved clinical result associated with the ITA graft is dependent on the superior late patency rates with this conduit, and thus on the surgeon's technical skill as well as the ITA's inherent resistance to atherosclerosis. The ITA graft should be used for as many anastomoses as possible. With the use of sequential, free, and bilateral grafts in a study[21] of 100 consecutive patients requiring multiple grafts, it was found possible to use ITA grafts for 70% of all anastomoses. With the increased use of the ITA graft, it might be anticipated that in the future even more favorable long-term results will be reported. However, the trend in patient selection is to choose sicker patients who have more risk factors for operative morbidity.[24] In these high risk patients, the need for the benefits conferred by ITA grafts wil be even greater. This modality should be used for as many grafts as possible and in every subgroup of patients.

REFERENCES

1. Kay HR, Korns ME, Flemma RJ, et al: Atherosclerosis of the internal mammary artery. *Ann Thorac Surg* 21:504–507, 1976.
2. Grondin CM, Campeau L, Lesperance J, et al: Comparison of the late changes in internal mammary artery and saphenous vein grafts in two consecutive series of patients 10 years after operation. *Circulation* 70:I-208–I-212, 1984.
3. Campeau L, Enjalbert M, Lesperance J, et al: Atherosclerosis and late closure of aortocoronary saphenous vein grafts: Sequential angiographic studies at 2 weeks, 1 year, 5 to 7 years, and 10 to 12 years after surgery. *Circulation* 68:II-1–II-7, 1983.
4. Zeff RH, Kongtahworn C, Iannone LA, et al: Internal mammary artery versus saphenous vein graft to the left anterior descending coronary artery: Prospective randomized study with 10-year follow-up. *Ann Thorac Surg* 45:533–536, 1988.

5. Schuster EH, Griffith LS, Bulkley BH, et al: Preponderance of acute proximal left anterior descending coronary arterial lesions in fatal myocardial infarction: A clinicopathologic study. *Am J Cardiol* 47:1189–1196, 1981.

6. Loop FD, Lytle BW, Cosgrove DM, et al: Influence of the internal-mammary-artery graft on 10-year survival and other cardiac events. *N Engl J Med* 314:1–6, 1986.

7. Okies JE, Page US, Bigelow JC, et al: The left internal mammary artery: The graft of choice. *Circulation* 70:I-213–I-221, 1984.

8. Cameron A, Kemp HG Jr, Green GE: Bypass surgery with the internal mammary artery graft: 15 year follow-up. *Circulation* 74:III-30–III-36, 1986.

9. Acinapura AJ, Rose DM, Jacobowitz IJ, et al: Internal mammary artery bypass grafting: Influence on recurrent angina and survival in 2,100 patients. *Ann Thorac Surg* 49:186–191, 1989.

10. Cameron A, Green GE: Unpublished data.

11. Cameron A, Davis KB, Green GE, et al: Clinical implications of internal mammary artery bypass grafts: The Coronary Artery Surgery Study experience. *Circulation* 77:815–819, 1988.

12. Cosgrove DM, Loop FD, Saunders CL, et al: Should coronary arteries with less than fifty percent stenosis be bypassed? *J Thorac Cardiovasc Surg* 82:520–530, 1981.

13. Lytle BW, Cosgrove DM, Saltus GL, et al: Multivessel coronary revascularization without saphenous vein: Long-term results of bilateral internal mammary artery grafting. *Ann Thorac Surg* 36:540–547, 1983.

14. Galbut DL, Traad EA, Dorman MJ, et al: Twelve-year experience with bilateral internal mammary artery grafts. *Ann Thorac Surg* 40:264–270, 1985.

15. Huddleston CB, Stoney WS, Alford WC Jr, et al: Internal mammary artery grafts: Technical factors influencing patency. *Ann Thorac Surg* 42:543–549, 1986.

16. Johnson WD, Brenowitz JB, Kayser KL: Factors influencing long-term (10-year to 15-year) survival after a successful coronary artery bypass operation. *Ann Thorac Surg* 48:19–25, 1989.

17. Fiore AC, Naunheim KS, Dean P, et al: Results of internal thoracic artery grafting over 15 years: Single vs. double grafts. *Ann Thorac Surg* 49:202–208, 1990.

18. Cheanvechai C, Irarrazaval MJ, Loop FD, et al: Aorta-coronary bypass grafting with the internal mammary artery. *J Thorac Cardiovasc Surg* 70:278–281, 1975.

19. Loop FD, Lytle BW, Cosgrove DM, et al: Free (aorta-coronary) internal mammary artery graft. *J Thorac Cardiovasc Surg* 92:827–831, 1986.

20. Sauvage LR, Wu HD, Kowalsky TE, et al: Healing basis and surgical techniques for complete revascularization of the left ventricle using only the internal mammary arteries. *Ann Thorac Surg* 42:449–465, 1986.

21. Green GE, Sosa JA, Cameron A: Prospective study of feasibility of routine use of multiple internal mammary artery anastomoses. *J Cardiovasc Surg* 30:643–647, 1989.

22. Tector AJ, Schmahl TM, Canino VR: Expanding the use of the internal mammary artery to improve patency in coronary artery bypass grafting. *J Thorac Cardiovasc Surg* 91:9–16, 1986.

23. Hodgson JM, Singh AK, Drew TM, et al: Coronary flow reserve provided by sequential internal mammary artery grafts. *J Am Coll Cardiol* 7:32–37, 1986.

24. Christakis GT, Ivanov J, Weisel RD, et al: The changing pattern of coronary artery bypass surgery. *Circulation* 80:I-151–I-161, 1989.

CHAPTER 6

Sternotomy Incision, Mobilization, and Routing of ITA Grafts

GEORGE E. GREEN

INCISION

Median sternotomy is the preferred incision for coronary bypass surgery and for mobilization of the internal thoracic arteries (ITAs). To avoid healing problems, meticulous attention must be paid to minimizing trauma to skin, subcutaneous tissue, fascia, periosteum, and bone.

Healing of the incision depends upon vascularity. Blood vessels of the region flow from lateral to medial. Midline anastomoses are tenuous. A precise midline incision preserves vascularity and enhances the stability of sternal closure by affording equal widths of bone for apposition. The best guide to the midline is the decussation of the pectoral and rectus muscles. Cautery, an invaluable aid to hemostasis, should be used with precision and restraint. Coagulation should be limited to the minimum depth required for hemostasis. Skin and subcutaneous fat should be divided by scalpel. Cautery should be used in pinpoint fashion. Application of optimum tension will define the fascia of the decussation of pectoral and rectus muscles. These may be divided either with a knife or with low-intensity coagulating current of the electrocautery. The notch of the manubrium is defined. The transverse cervical veins just above the notch are displaced cephalad. The interclavicular ligament is defined and divided. Beginning at this time and continuing frequently throughout the operation, the wound is irrigated with 50-ml aliquots of an antibiotic solution containing 500 mg of vancomycin per 1,000 ml of normal saline. One liter of this solution is used during the operation. The periosteum of the sternum is divided in the midline. An oscillating saw is used to divide the sternum along this midline incision. The saw blade must be sharp enough and the oscillation fast enough to divide bone without stripping periosteum.

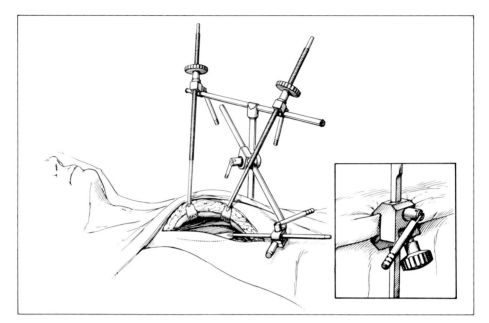

FIGURE 6–1 A self-retaining sternal retractor clamps to the table over the drapes.

MOBILIZATION AND ROUTING OF ITA GRAFTS

A self-retaining retractor to elevate the sternum facilitates dissection of the ITAs. The base of the retractor is fixed to the side of the operating table. A model that clamps over the surgical drapes is most convenient (Fig. 6–1). The vertical bar of the retractor is at the level of the upper arm. In patients of large habitus, the bar can press on the arm. If the patient's arm is in contact with the bar, the surgeon must draw the patient's shoulder away from the retractor bar. Compression of the arm against the bar where the radial nerve curves laterally around the humerous can cause palsy. If surgical drapes become wet or if electrical grounding of the cautery unit is inadequate, pressure of the arm on the bar can result in an electrical burn. It is usually most convenient to mobilize the left ITA before mobilizing the right, and immediately after the sternotomy incision. The distal of the two retractor rakes is placed at the xiphi-sternal joint. The sternum is elevated sufficiently to place tension on the mediastinal fascia connecting the pericardium to the posterior periosteum of the sternum and the diaphragm to the posterior rectus sheath. Additional tension is applied with countertraction. Low-intensity coagulating current is used to divide these fasciae. The sternum can then be elevated further. The second rake of the retractor is applied at the level of the sternoclavicular joint. Traction here relieves tension on the xiphi-sternal rake, which is elevated further.

The parietal pleura can be reflected off the internal thoracic fascia sufficiently to permit dissection of the ITAs. However, exposure of the ITA at the thoracic inlet is greatly facilitated by displacing the apex of the lung, which is best done after opening the pleura. Furthermore, at the end of the operation, covering the heart and grafts and filling the retrosternal space with vascularized tissue require suturing pleuropericardial tissues over the heart and grafts. Such shifting of tissues can best be done after widely dividing both pleural membranes.

The left pleura is divided close to the chest wall from diaphragm to thoracic inlet. The left lung is displaced. The medial and lateral internal thoracic veins and the ITA are usually visible and palpable. Pleura, fascia, and muscle are divided just medial to the medial internal thoracic vein. They are reflected laterally off the ITA and its veins. The medial vein is grasped and used as a tractor to separate the vascular pedicle from the chest wall. A thin cautery blade is a helpful dissector. When there is sufficient separation of vascular pedicle from chest wall, the forceps is placed between the pedicle and the chest wall to continue traction. The most important points of fixation of the pedicle to the chest wall are branches of the ITA and tributaries of its veins. The arterial branches, the anterior intercostals, arise in the middle of each interspace and bifurcate into a superior and an inferior branch. They anastomose with corresponding branches of the posterior intercostal arteries from the descending thoracic aorta (Fig. 6–2). There are additional anastomoses with branches of the thoracoacromial and lateral costal arteries. The thoracoacromial branches are an anterior collateral supply. They penetrate the pectoral muscles to reach the chest wall. The lateral costal branches course just beneath the pleura in a midlateral position. When the anterior intercostal arteries are divided from the ITA, there is copious collateral flow to the anterior rami, the distribution system to the sternum.

Large vascular branches, 1 mm or more in diameter, are best secured with small hemoclips. These larger branches have sufficient flow so that heat is dissipated and they are not readily sealed by a low current. Common sites of large intercostal branches are the second and third interspaces. Sufficient length of these vessels should be developed so that neither the ITA nor the superior or inferior divisions of its anterior intercostal branches are damaged. If the internal intercostal muscle and the fascia covering it are not disrupted, the terminal branches will not be jeopardized. Other structures which bind the vascular pedicle to the chest wall are intercostal nerve branches, lymphatics, and the fascia that connects them. These structures, when under appropriate tension, are readily divided by low-intensity coagulating current.

Previous costochondral inflammation (most commonly due to severe trauma) causes the fascia connecting internal thoracic blood vessels, lymphatics, and nerves to become densely fibrotic, binding the ITA closely to the chest wall. Dissection then becomes difficult. To avoid ITA injury, perichondrium may have to be stripped from the costal cartilage, and if separation of the ITA from the internal intercostal muscle is difficult, muscle may have to be included with the vascular pedicle. The terminal intercostal vasculature is then prone to disruption, and sternal vascularity may be impaired. When such inflammation involves both sides of the chest, use of both ITAs may be unwise.

Abnormalities of skeletal development increase the difficulty of ITA mobilization but do not preclude it. In pectus excavatum the ITA is displaced later-

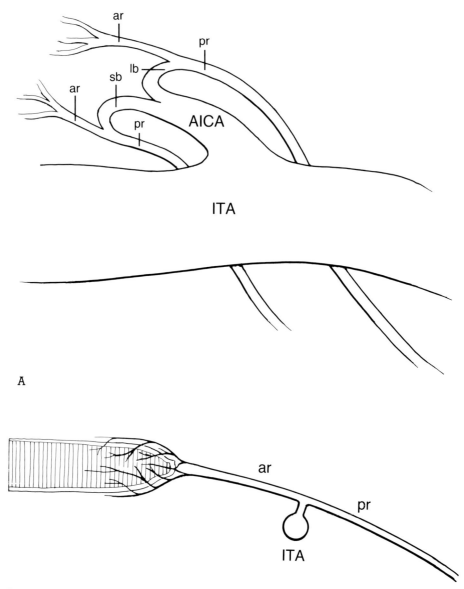

FIGURE 6–2 **A:** An anterior intercostal artery (AICA) arises from the ITA in each intercostal space. Each AICA divides into a superior and an inferior branch (SB, IB). Each branch divides into anterior and posterior rami (ar, pr). **B:** Each anterior ramus supplies branches to the anterior and posterior periosteum and the marrow of the sternum.

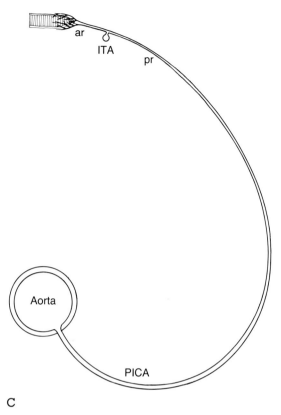

C

FIGURE 6–2 Continued **C:** The posterior ramus anastomoses with the corresponding ramus of the posterior intercostal artery (PICA).

ally. It usually has a good caliber. Despite the lateral displacement, adequate exposure usually can be obtained.

Exposure of the ITA can be difficult in patients who have a high-vaulted chest. The high arch of the chest opposite the side of dissection obstructs the surgeons' line of vision. Forceful depression of this side of the chest may be necessary. The area of most difficult exposure is the second interspace, where the arch is highest.

Rigidity of ribs and costal cartilages increases the possibility of rib fracture or costochondral dislocation. Costochondral dislocation seriously impairs spreading of the sternum and results in poor exposure. Rib fractures cause postoperative discomfort that interferes with ventilation.

Dissection above the first intercostal space enters the domain of the phrenic nerve (Fig. 6–3). It passes close behind the ITA and internal thoracic vein. Division of the internal thoracic vein just before it enters the subclavian facilitates identification of the nerve and exposure and mobilization of the proximal portion of the ITA. The phrenic nerve is sometimes closely adherent to the ITA. Dissection in the fat pad of this area will reveal arterial branches from

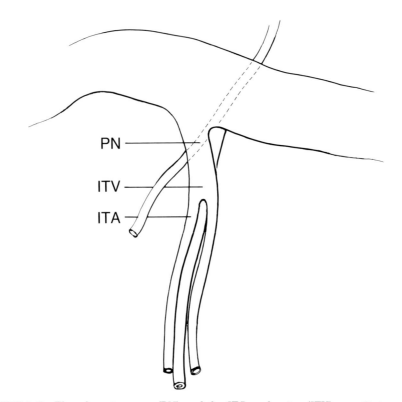

FIGURE 6–3 The phrenic nerve (PN) and the ITA and veins (ITV) constitute a neuro-vascular bundle.

the ITA to the thymus and the strap muscles. Occasionally, the inferior thyroid or lateral costal arteries arise from the ITA here. Arterial branches are mobilized and divided. Fascial strands binding the phrenic nerve to the ITA are divided. The phrenic nerve is displaced medially away from the ITA. The fat pad lateral to the ITA contains lymphatic vessels. It is divided by electrocautery or secured with hemoclips and divided with scissors. If the phrenic nerve has not been definitively identified, low-intensity electrocoagulation is safest. Neuromuscular blockade from anesthesia is rarely profound enough to prevent diaphragmatic stimulation by electrical contact with phrenic nerve fibrils. Following full mobilization, the ITA will fall medially and posteriorly to parallel the phrenic nerve. It will be well medial to the upper lobe of the lung. Expansion of the lung can then never distract the arterial graft from the heart.

Although the ITA usually arises from the first portion of the subclavian artery, opposite the vertebral artery or thyrocervical trunk, it sometimes arises much more medially or laterally. When it arises very medially, it is subject to damage because it may not be covered by the internal thoracic vein. If the electrocautery makes direct contact with the ITA, severe damage is incurred. Spasm always occurs. Thrombosis can ensue. If the injury has not been severe enough to cause thrombosis, late stricture may ensue. When cau-

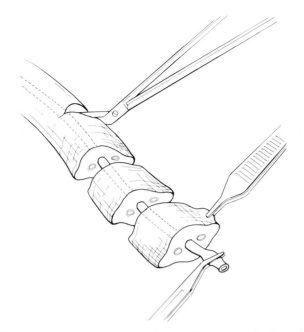

FIGURE 6–4 Transection of extraneous tissues increases the length and mobility of the ITA pedicle.

tery injures the ITA, the artery should not be used as a pedicled graft. It can be transected, excluding the site of injury, and used as a free graft.

After the left ITA has been mobilized from its origin to the sixth intercostal space, it is divided. I prefer to divide it just proximal to its bifurcation into the sixth intercostal (musculophrenic) and superior epigastric branches. Ligation which leaves these branches in continuity contributes to the vascularity of the chest wall and the upper abdominal wall. It also affords the larger area of the ITA proper for anastomosis.

If, because of chest wall inflammation, mobilization of a narrow pedicle containing only ITAs and internal thoracic veins was not possible, adherent tissues, pleura, transverse thoracic fascia, and transverse thoracic muscle should be transected in stepladder fashion to increase the length and mobility of the graft (Fig. 6–4). They are not necessary to the nutrition of the graft.[1]

The pericardium is opened from the diaphragmatic reflection out to the apex of the heart and up to the distal ascending aorta. If the ITA is to be used as a pedicled graft, this pleuropericardial flap is elevated. An incision anterior to the phrenic nerve is made in the pleuropericardial flap if the pedicle is to be brought to the anterior surface of the heart (Fig. 6–5). The pedicle is laid on the anterior surface of the heart, and the length to the area of proposed anastomosis is marked on the pedicle. If the ITA graft is to be brought to the posterior surface of the heart, length can be saved by drawing it through an incision posterior to the phrenic nerve.

Regardless of the degree of myocardial ischemia, effective anesthesia emphasizing constant afterload reduction (vasodilation) and avoiding excessive

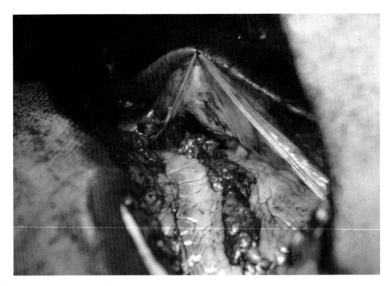

FIGURE 6-5 The left ITA is brought through the pleuropericardial fold near the phrenic nerve. (Figure 6-5 appears in color after chapter 8.)

preload (hypervolemia) usually maintains a stable hemodynamic state. This is indicated most importantly by the appearance of the heart. The ventricles should not be distended or sluggish. Corollary findings are stability of the electrocardiogram (ECG), mixed venous oxygen saturation, and cardiac output. If anesthesia has maintained systolic blood pressure in a relatively low range (90–100 mm), cardiac appearance, ECG, mixed venous oxygen saturation, and cardiac output are almost always satisfactory.

If the hemodynamic state is not satisfactory, heparin is administered and circulatory support is started. If, as is usual, the hemodynamic situation is satisfactory, the right ITA is mobilized. A frequent difference between the right and left sides is that the right internal thoracic vein usually drains into the superior vena cava, not the subclavian vein. The proximal 3 cm of the right ITA is usually not shielded by the vein and is subject to injury. The right ITA should be mobilized as fully as the left.

Routing of Right ITA Grafts

If the right ITA is to be used as a graft to the posterior descending artery, it is allowed to lie parallel to the right phrenic nerve until it reaches the level of the inferior pulmonary vein. Here it is drawn through an incision anterior to the phrenic nerve. If the right ITA is to be used as a graft to the left side of the heart, it is drawn through a proximal incision in the pleuropericardial fold just anterior to the phrenic nerve and the superior vena cava. Alternatively, the entire pleuropericardial fold can be divided down to the superior vena cava. The arterial pedicle is brought across the aorta, just proximal to the origin of the innominate artery and across the main pulmonary artery to the interventricular groove. When the right ITA is used as a graft to branches of the circumflex artery, I usually find that the route anterior to the aorta is also the shortest. Bringing the right ITA through the transverse sinus usually requires more length because of sharp angulation going into the transverse sinus. These in vivo observations differ from Van der Salm et al.'s postmortem observations.[2] When heart-lung bypass has been terminated, all pedicle grafts should have ample length. If the heart pulls on the pedicle with each beat, the length is certainly inadequate. Adequacy of the length is confirmed by displacing the graft 1–2 cm medially and laterally. There should be no pull on the anastomosis with such displacement. Inadequate length will cause fibrotic stricture of the anastomosis or of the graft, or both. Inadequacy of the length must be corrected by converting the pedicled graft to a free graft. Although closing the sternum diminishes the distance from the subclavian origin of the graft to the coronary anastomosis, upright posture increases it. Pedicled grafts must manifest ample length prior to closure of the chest.

REFERENCES

1. Sauvage LR, Wu HD, Kowalsky TE, et al: Healing basis and surgical techniques for complete revascularization of the left ventricle using only the internal mammary arteries. *Ann Thorac Surg* 42:449–465, 1986.
2. Van der Salm TJ, Chowdhary S, Okike ON: Internal mammary artery grafts: The shortest route to the coronary arteries. *Ann Thorac Surg* 47:421–427, 1989.

CHAPTER **7**

Cannulations, Heart-Lung Bypass, and Cardioplegia

GEORGE E. GREEN

Cannulations, conduct of heart-lung bypass, and delivery of cardioplegia are significantly different for coronary surgery than for other types of cardiac surgery. The ideal site for aortic cannulation is at the distal pericardial reflection. This allows maximum choice for placement of cross-clamp and proximal anastomoses. However, atherosclerosis of the aorta is frequent in patients with coronary disease. An area free of atherosclerosis should be chosen for cannulation to avoid atheroembolism. Prominent vascularity of aortic adventitia suggests atherosclerosis, as does fixation of the adventitia to the aortic wall. Palpable induration of the wall is definitive but requires low aortic pressure to be discerned. Reduction of pressure can readily be achieved by temporary venous inflow occlusion. An incision through an atherosclerotic wall results in surprisingly little bleeding. In such instances, it is best to close that aortotomy site and move to another site for cannulation. In rare instances when no satisfactory site can be found for cannulation of the ascending aorta, the aortic arch or the femoral arteries should be explored.

Venous cannulation for coronary surgery should allow maximum mobility of the heart so that optimal exposure of all coronary segments can be obtained. Single venous cannulation allows more mobility than double venous cannulation. Too large a venous cannula is an impediment. I prefer a No. 40 French cannula with sufficient holes so that the distal end of the cannula is in the inferior vena cavae just below the eustachian valve and several ports drain the right atrium.

A large (No. 28 French), well-positioned ventricular vent is extremely helpful. Manipulation of the heart to explore coronary segments, and manipulation of the aorta when performing proximal anastomoses, cause aortic insufficiency with significant frequency. A large, well-functioning vent facilitates manipulation of the heart and prevents myocardial injury by preventing distention. I prefer to introduce the ventricular vent from the interatrial groove rather

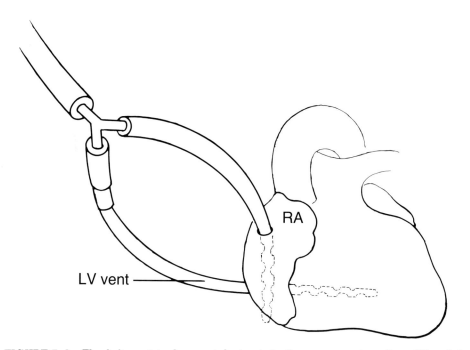

FIGURE 7–1 The left ventricular vent drains into the venous return line. LV = left ventricle; RA = right atrium

than from the superior pulmonary vein. Passage through the mitral orifice into the left ventricle may require manual guidance from the oblique sinus. The position of the cannula is maintained by tightening a tourniquet around a mattress suture placed in the tissues of the interatrial groove. The vent cannula is secured to the tourniquet. Those who avoid the use of a ventricular vent contend that it can be a source of air embolism. This is avoided by fibrillating the heart or keeping the heart full when it is beating. When fibrillation is prolonged, blood temperature should be reduced to 28°C. At this temperature, fibrillation is so fine that little energy is expended by the myocardium. Maintenance of perfusion pressure at about 80 mm affords ideal nutrition to the vented, fibrillating heart.[1,2] Induced fibrillation with the ventricles vented and cooled affords excellent myocardial protection and excellent conditions for scrutinizing the anatomy and pathology of coronary segments.

The vent can be connected either to pump suction or to the venous gravity drainage line (Fig. 7–1). I prefer the latter.

With the ventricles fibrillating, the coronary arteries are inspected visually and by palpation. Angiography is the criterion of sites of critical obstruction, but appearance and pliability are the criteria of where to place the arteriotomy. An area at least 1 cm beyond the most distal site of atherosclerotic change should be chosen. The reasons are three:

1. Endarterectomy can be avoided. The most common reason cited for performing endarterectomy is "necessity." This situation usually is caused by attempting arteriotomy through an atherosclerotic wall. The risks of

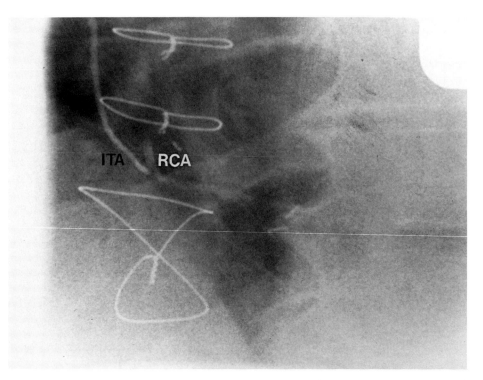

FIGURE 7–2 ITA anastomosis to an atherosclerotic right coronary artery resulted in stricture 18 months after the operation.

infarction and mortality incurred by endarterectomy exceed those of simple bypass.[3] Endarterectomy puts both proximal and distal flow at risk because of the thrombogenic nature of the endarterectomy bed and the possibility of loose intimal flaps at its termination.

2. Even if endarterectomy is avoided, healing of anastomoses to atherosclerotic arteries increases likelihood of stricture (Fig. 7–2).

3. If arteriotomy is unduly close to an atherosclerotic plaque, progression of atherosclerosis may encompass and narrow the area of anastomosis (Fig. 7–3).

Angiography frequently fails to indicate areas of early atherosclerosis because dilatation can be concurrent with atheromatous thickening. Such thickening is apparent as palpable induration. It is accompanied by an inflammatory reaction in the adventitia marked by increased vascularity and adhesion of epicardium to adventitia. This is usually apparent before arteriotomy is begun. If arteriotomy in such areas is begun, it should not be completed. A more distal site should be chosen.

The process of arteriotomy should be gradual and progressive. Epicardium should be divided first, then adventitia, and finally media and intima. In normal areas, the intima is very thin and closely adherent to the media. In areas of atherosclerotic change, smooth muscle cells pass through gaps in the inter-

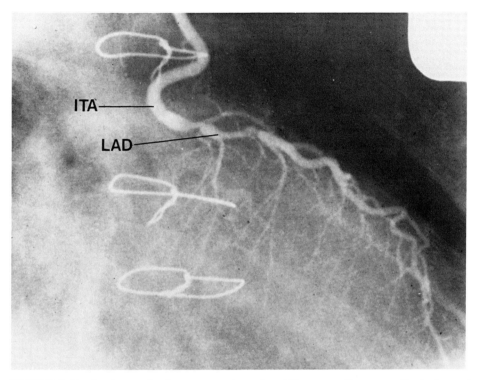

FIGURE 7-3 Angiography for recurrent angina (15 years after operation) showed progression of atherosclerosis to and just beyond the site of the ITA-LAD anastomosis. The original anastomosis was placed close to an atherosclerotic plaque because the LAD beyond it was covered by heart muscle. Myotomy and more distal anastomosis should have been done originally and were necessary 15 years later. The distal LAD was much larger than was suggested by angiogram.

nal elastic membrane into the intima and proliferate. Monocytes invade, accumulate lipid, and become foam cells. From 10- to 50-fold thickening of intima results. When such thickening is encountered, arteriotomy should be stopped. High magnification (8×) is a great help in the process of arteriotomy. It is crucial in choosing more distal sites for arteriotomy and in performing anastomosis to smaller distal vessels. The undesirable choice of endarterectomy is often explained as the only way that bypass can be achieved. Endarterectomy is the only way bypass can be achieved without high magnification. With no or low magnification, patency of grafts to coronary segments less than 1.5 mm is unacceptable.[4] With high magnification, consistent wide patency of such anastomoses is obtained.[5]

Ventricular fibrillation can be used very effectively as the mode of cardioplegia during anastomosis. Temporary local occlusion proximal and distal to the arteriotomy is required. Fine Potts bulldog clamps or temporary local occlusion ligatures can be used (Fig. 7-4A,B). During such anastomoses, it is crucial that the ventricular vent not be displaced into the atrium. As the heart is manipulated, the ventricle can be drawn away from the tip of the venting

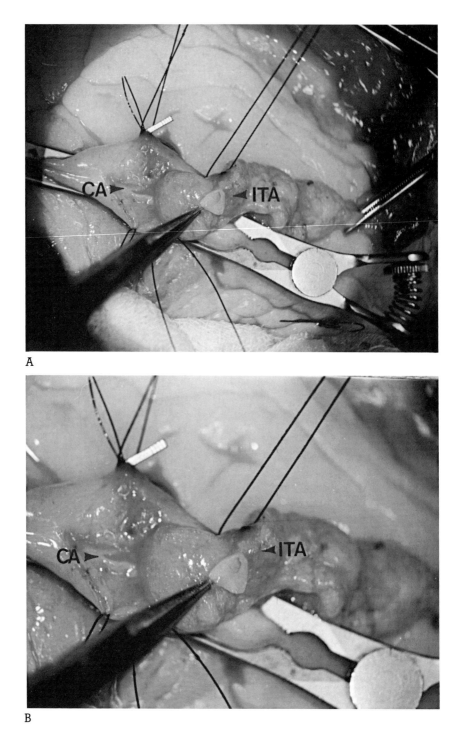

FIGURE 7–4 **A:** Local occlusion with fine Potts clamps allows anastomosis with the heart fibrillating. Photographed through a microscope at 3×. **B:** 6×.

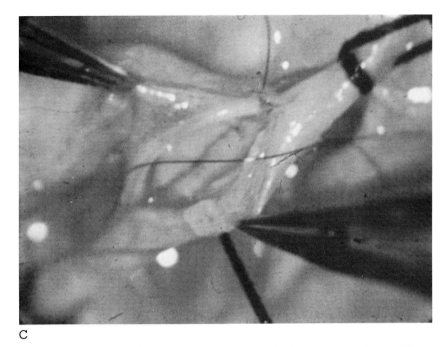

C

FIGURE 7–4 Continued   C: Local occlusion can also be accomplished with tempo-rary ligatures. Photographed through a microscope at 8×.

cannula. If the vent is displaced into the left atrium, even a small degree of aortic insufficiency can cause ventricular distention. With surgical awareness, distention is readily recognized. It is resolved by repositioning the vent. Pro-longed ventricular distention is very damaging and must be avoided.

Optimal exposure of the circumflex artery and its branches requires bring-ing the lateral surface of the ventricle anterior and medial until it is in the midline. This can be achieved readily when both pleural spaces are opened. Traction on the posterior pericardium lateral to the left pulmonary veins will bring the lateral surface of the ventricle forward. The anterior surface of the ventricle is rolled under the right side of the sternum and into the open right pleural space[6] (Fig. 7–5). This rotation can distort the aortic annulus and cause aortic insufficiency. A well-functioning vent prevents distention of the ventricle, but if the aortic insufficiency is large, perfusion pressure will fall. It is not desirable for perfusion pressure to be less than 70 mm when the ventricles are fibrillating. Aortic insufficiency can be terminated by cross-clamping the aorta. If clamp time is more than 20 minutes, cold cardioplegia solution should be administered. Infusion into the arteriotomy alone is not sufficient to protect the entire myocardium, but cardioplegia cannot be admin-istered effectively into the aorta with insufficiency. The aortic clamp is re-moved, the heart is returned to a neutral position, and the traction on the pericardium is released. The aorta is then clamped for the delivery of cardi-oplegia solution. The clamp is placed as far from the aortic annulus as possible and at a right angle to the aorta. This position minimizes the incidence of

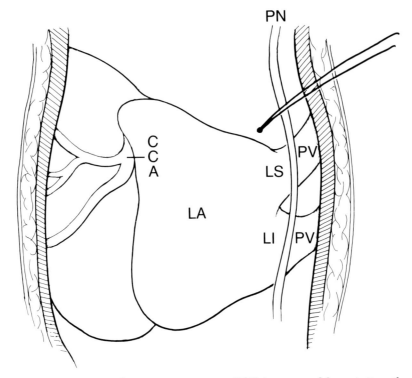

FIGURE 7-5 The circumflex coronary artery CCA is exposed by rotating the apex of the heart into the right pleural space. PN = phrenic nerve; LSPV = left superior pulmonary vein; LIPV = left inferior pulmonary vein; LA = left atrium.

aortic insufficiency due to clamping. There are many ways of delivering cardioplegia solution.[7] I prefer a thin-walled No. 14 needle. The solution is infused at a rate of 400 ml per minute, a volume that approaches normal coronary flow. Smaller volumes of flow do not achieve homogeneous delivery of solution. One liter of solution is administered. If stenoses are multiple and severe, aortic pressure may become excessive, with delivery of 400 ml per minute. In such situations, the rate of administration is reduced, but 2 liters may have to be infused before homogeneous cooling is achieved. The needle is removed from the aorta. When cardioplegia is administered, arterial flow is reduced so that all venous return is readily removed from the right atrium. Maintaining an empty heart is important in keeping the heart cold. The heart is repositioned, again exposing the circumflex artery and its branches. The myocardium is surrounded with cold laparotomy pads. Anastomosis to the circumflex artery or its branches is then performed.

There are occasional patients in whom, despite placement of the cross-clamp transversely across the distal ascending aorta, distortion of the aortic annulus occurs and causes aortic insufficiency, preventing effective delivery of cardioplegia. This is manifested by low tension in the ascending aorta and rapid reflux of cardioplegia solution through the left ventricular vent. There are three potential ways to proceed.

1. Aortic clamp time can be limited to 20 minutes and reperfusion allowed for 5- to 10-minute intervals between clamp applications.
2. Retrograde cardioplegia can be administered by the coronary sinus.[8]
3. The ascending aorta can be opened and both coronary ostia cannulated with loose-fitting silastic cannulas. Then 400 ml of cardioplegia solution per minute can be administered by a Y connector attached to the cardioplegia line. I use selective coronary cannulation whenever coronary surgery is combined with aortic valve surgery and when aortic cross-clamping causes severe aortic insufficiency in mitral valve surgery. I have had no complications from leaving loose-fitting silastic cannulas in the coronary ostia and delivering 1 liter of cardioplegia solution at a rate of 400 ml/min every 15 minutes. Prior to learning that cannulation of coronary ostia with oversized cannulas could cause late ostial stenosis, I used snugly-fitting cannulas and did observe instances of late ostial stenosis.

Composition of the optimal cardioplegia solution is speculative. The solution I have used (with an overall mortality of 1–2% for coronary surgery, a myocardial infarction rate of 1–2%, and the need for intra-aortic balloon pump assistance in less than 1% of cases) is a cold, oxygenated, crystalloid solution. It is composed of 1,000 ml of 5% dextrose containing 25 mEq of sodium bicarbonate, 10 mEq of potassium chloride, and 1 mg of verapamil (for the first liter only). The solution is cooled to 4°C and oxygenated by injecting 100 ml of oxygen in each liter of solution. The large volumes of crystalloid solution delivered are eliminated by induction of diuresis or by in-line dialysis.

When saphenous vein grafts are performed, 200–300 ml of additional cardioplegia solution is administered through the vein graft at the completion of each anastomosis. This tests the integrity of the anastomosis and maintains cooling of the myocardium. When internal thoracic artery (ITA) grafts are done, 200–300 ml of cardioplegia solution is administered into each arteriotomy (Fig. 7–6a–c). To test the integrity of ITA anastomoses, perfusion pressure is raised to 100 mm mean by administration of phenylephrine. When the ITA pedicle is unclamped, there should be prompt filling of the coronary distribution, with ample fullness of coronary branches and the ITA. Bleeding from ITA side branches is controlled with point cautery or hemoclips. Bleeding from the anastomosis is controlled with an additional stitch. The pedicle is again clamped, and perfusion pressure is allowed to drop to its usual level.

When coronary anastomoses are completed, the aortic cross-clamp, if used, is removed. The heart, if fibrillating, is defibrillated. The blood is rewarmed. During rewarming, proximal vein anastomoses, if needed, are performed. Pacemaker wires and pleural drainage tubes are placed. Rewarming is facilitated by the highest possible pump flow. Water temperature is kept 7–10°C above blood temperature but not above 40°C. Ventilation is resumed. Rewarming is continued to a core (rectal or nasopharyngeal) temperature of 35°C. Premature discontinuation of heart-lung bypass will leave tissues cold, vasoconstricted, and acidotic, the prelude to an unstable postoperative course. Moreover, blood platelet function is seriously impaired during hypothermia.

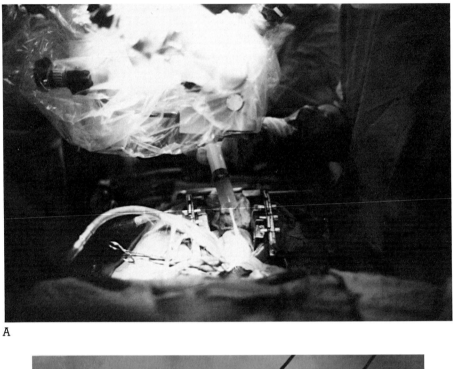

A

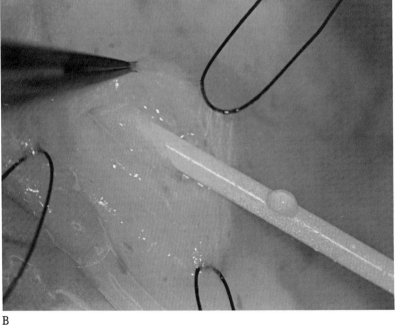

B

FIGURE 7–6 Delivery of cardioplegia into each arteriotomy before ITA anastomosis maintains cooling. **A:** Distant view of the microscope and the infusion. **B:** Antegrade infusion photographed through a microscope at 8×.

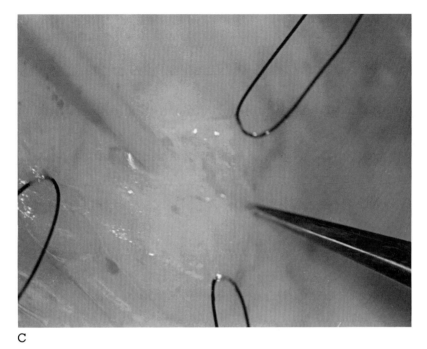

C

FIGURE 7–6 Continued   C: Retrograde infusion photographed through a microscope at 8×.

When core temperature is 35°C and blood chemistries are normal, the patient is ready to be weaned from bypass. With maximum pump flow, mean perfusion pressure should be 70 mm Hg. If pressure is less than 70 mm Hg, it is raised by progressive infusion of norepinephrine. As the pressure is being adjusted, the left ventricular cannula is withdrawn into the left atrium. The venous return line is progressively occluded, and pump flow is reduced. Blood is infused into the patient until the heart appears full. Bypass is then discontinued. Left atrial pressure is measured by opening the left atrial vent to air. If left atrial pressure is unduly high, blood is aspirated from the left atrial cannula. If left atrial pressure is unduly low, blood is infused from the oxygenator until the height of the column of blood in the left atrial cannula is about 15 cm (approximately 15 mm Hg). If the right ventricle becomes distended during the infusion of blood, infusion is discontinued before left atrial pressure reaches 15 mm Hg. Usually heart action appears homogeneously vigorous, mixed venous oxygen saturation is about 80%, and the cardiac index is about 3 liters/min. If heart action seems poor, or if the mixed venous oxygen saturation or cardiac index is abnormally low, circulatory support is reinstituted. After maximum pump flow is achieved, mean arterial pressure is again raised to 100 mm Hg by infusion of phenylephrine. The purpose of raising arterial pressure is to be sure that any residual air is moved through the coronary arteries. Decompressing both sides of the heart while raising perfusion pressure affords optimal nutrition to the myocardium. After several minutes, the right atrial cannula is clamped so that full blood flow passes through the lungs. Residual air bubbles are a relatively common and easily remediable cause of depressed cardiac action in the immediate postbypass period. Circulatory support using the left atrial cannula and maintaining high mean perfusion pressure (100 mm) is continued for several more minutes. Circulatory support is discontinued. Blood pressure is maintained above 100 mm systolic by adjustment of intravascular volume and administration of norepinephrine. At a systolic pressure of 100 mm and physiological ranges of right and left atrial pressure, heart action should appear satisfactory, and mixed venous oxygen saturation and cardiac index should be in a physiological range. Occasionally, despite normal parameters, large amounts (more than 10 µg) of norepinephrine is necessary to maintain systolic blood pressure at 100 mm. If peripheral arterial resistance is below normal, the need for levofed is not of adverse significance. If peripheral resistance is increased and cardiac output is low, myocardial insufficiency exists. Despite much talk about "reperfusion injury," the injury is basically a result of ischemia. If the arterial obstruction was relieved by the surgery, injury was caused by one or two aspects of the procedure. If aortic cross-clamping was employed, inadequate delivery of cardioplegia and inadequate cooling were the probable causes. If ventricular fibrillation was employed, inadequate venting or inadequate perfusion pressure were probably to blame.

Minor injury to the left ventricle, and minor or moderate injury to the right ventricle, can usually be managed by careful adjustment of intravascular volume and judicious use of vasopressors and/or inotropes.

Profound impairment restricted to the right ventricle is rare. It is best managed by right heart assistance. This can be achieved with right atrial and pulmonary artery cannulas bridged by a centrifugal pump.

Moderate left ventricular impairment can be alleviated by the use of an intra-aortic balloon pump. This can be inserted through either the femoral artery or the ascending aorta. Patients with small iliofemoral systems, notably small women, may develop limb-threatening ischemia after transfemoral placement. This is more common with the percutaneous than with the open mode of insertion.[9] In such instances and in patients with serious iliofemoral disease, I prefer to insert the intra-aortic balloon pump through the ascending aorta at the aortic cannulation site. After the patient is weaned from bypass, the aortic cannula is removed and the purse string sutures are tied around the balloon pump catheter. The catheter is brought outside the pericardium between the right pericardial fold and the lung. It exits at the lowest angle of the incision. Routine closure of the chest, as described below, is performed. Return to the operating room will be necessary for removal, but this is preferable to the alternative method of leaving a long sleeve of prosthetic material on the aorta.

If, despite the use of the intra-aortic balloon pump, left ventricular function is so profoundly impaired that weaning from bypass cannot be achieved, a left ventricular assist device can be employed. The simplest method is to bridge the left atrial cannula to the aortic cannula with a centrifugal pump.[10]

Rarely, both right and left ventricular function can be so profoundly impaired that biventricular assist is necessary. This can be accomplished with two centrifugal pumps combining both right and left heart assist.

After discontinuation of heart-lung bypass, protamine is administered. Protamine can cause serious impairment of myocardial contractility, most often manifested by marked distention of the right ventricle. When impairment is profound, I have discontinued the use of protamine and administered no more of it. In these instances, I have not encountered critical bleeding despite incomplete administration of the calculated dose of protamine. Indeed, activated clotting time has often been in a normal range.

In the usual situation, when protamine administration has been completed, blood clot formation should be evident. If no blood clot is discernible, a bleeding diathesis has occurred. Such diatheses are marked by inadequate platelet function and fibrinolysis. Both are a reaction of blood to contact with the oxygenator. Fibrinolysis is due to activation of plasminogen to plasmin. Aminocaproic acid blocks the conversion of plasminogen to plasmin. Large doses can block the action of plasmin. When no clot is observed, I give 10 g of aminocaproic acid. Desmopressin (0.3 mg/kg) is given to enhance platelet activity. From 6 to 12 units of platelets are requested for transfusion. Closure of the chest incision then begins. If the right ITA has been brought through an incision in the right pleuropericardial fold at the level of the diaphragm, adequate pericardial drainage is present. If this incision has not been made, a 4-cm incision anterior to the phrenic nerve is placed at the level of the diaphragm. The pleuropericardial folds are closed over the heart and grafts with interrupted sutures. The right pericardial fat pad is brought medially and anteriorly over the pleuropericardial folds so that the retrosternal space is obliterated.[11] The wound is again irrigated with antibiotic solution. Residual blood in the pleural spaces is not aspirated. It is left to defibrinate so that it can be reinfused later. The chest wall is again inspected for bleeding from sites of ITA mobilization. This must be done at a systolic pressure of above 100 mm. Norepinephrine is administered as needed. Bleeding points are secured as necessary. Excessive use of cautery is avoided. The sternum is closed with stainless steel wires placed through the manubrium but around segments of the body of the sternum. One wire is placed in each interspace. I prefer closing fascia, subcutaneous tissue, and skin with interrupted, nonabsorbable sutures.

If there is still no evidence of blood clot, even if no unusual bleeding is observed, administration of blood platelets is warranted. I find this to be so in about 5% of patients.

Pleural drainage tubes are now connected to a reinfusion system.

SPECIAL CONSIDERATIONS IN REOPERATIONS

Reoperations comprise at least 10% of coronary surgical practice. The need for reoperation increases with the time after the previous surgery. Special problems with exposure of the heart and management of old grafts warrant attention.

If the heart is not separated from the chest wall by pericardium, pleuropericardial membranes, or lung, reopening the chest can damage the heart or grafts. Sternotomy is most safely done with an oscillating saw that can divide the anterior and then the posterior tables of the sternum separately.

If the heart or the grafts are adherent to the chest wall, traction on them is necessary. However, this can critically depress cardiac function, impair flow through nonsclerotic grafts, and embolize atheromatous debris from sclerotic grafts. Dissection is easier and safer if the heart is decompressed and assisted circulation is provided. This is accomplished by cannulation of the femoral vein and artery and use of the heart-lung machine.

The femoral vein and artery are exposed through an oblique incision in the inguinal fold. The femoral vein is isolated just above the saphenofemoral junction and mobilized for approximately 4 cm. The common femoral artery is isolated just above the profunda femoris branch for a similar distance. Heparin (4,000 units/kg) is administered. A vascular clamp is applied across the common femoral vein at the saphenofemoral junction. A tape is passed around the proximal end of the common femoral vein. It is then brought through a tourniquet. A vascular clamp is placed across the common femoral vein at the level of the tape. The anterior half of the common femoral vein is divided. A traction suture is placed in the middle of the proximal half of the venotomy. The proximal vascular clamp is removed. A No. 28 French drainage catheter is advanced from the venotomy to the right atrium. The tape is secured around the vein and cannula with the tourniquet. The distal common femoral artery is clamped just proximal to the profunda femoris. A tape and tourniquet are placed around the proximal common femoral artery. The anterior half of the common femoral artery is transected. A No. 20 French arterial cannula is introduced and secured with the tape and tourniquet. The venous and arterial cannulas are connected to the heart-lung machine, and circulatory support is begun. Flows are kept at a maximal level, usually in the range of 3 liters/min. Decompression of the heart is notable. Blood temperature is lowered to 28°C. Dissection of the heart and grafts from the chest wall continues. A self-retaining sternal retractor is helpful (see Fig. 6–1).

If an ITA graft was previously done, the lung is usually adherent to the parietal pleura. Dissection of the lung from the parietal pleura is begun at the level of the diaphragm and continued to the apex of the chest. Dissection should initially be extended well laterally, at least to the midaxillary line. As dissection is continued proximally, it moves from lateral to medial. Above the second intercostal space, the ITA may be encountered. It should be mobilized to its origin. This can be difficult, and the potential for damage to the ITA exists. If the artery is disrupted, catastrophic myocardial ischemia can ensue. If disruption occurs and cannot be readily bridged by an intravascular shunt, it is best to cannulate the distal segment with a 2-mm silastic cannula and perfuse it with arterial blood from the heart-lung machine. Saphenous vein grafts adherent to the chest wall usually become so thickened that disruption is unlikely. However, when such grafts are atherosclerotic, manipulation of them can cause irremediable embolization of atherosclerotic debris. Particular attention should be paid to minimizing manipulation of saphenous vein grafts. After the heart has been mobilized from the chest wall, it is progressively mobilized from the mediastinum until a left ventricular vent can be inserted in the area of the interatrial groove. The heart is stilled by electrical fibrillation. This facilitates complete mobilization with the least likelihood of trauma. A right atrial cannula is usually needed to obtain complete right heart decompression. It is bridged to the venous gravity drainage system.

Operation proceeds as described for primary operation, except for three caveats.

1. If cross-clamping of the ascending aorta is performed, flow through ITA grafts should be interrupted with vascular clamps. If occlusion of previous ITA grafts is not done, dry arteriotomies cannot be obtained. Also, there will be early washout of cardioplegia solution and rewarming of the myocardium. Lowering the perfusion temperature to 20°C will diminish the rewarming effect. Reducing perfusion pressure to 30 mm will help achieve a dry arteriotomy.

2. When the ascending aorta is clamped, I administer the first dose of cardioplegia solution as usual. Thereafter each sclerotic vein graft is divided proximal to its coronary anastomosis. The transected grafts are not secured by ligature until the ascending aorta has been unclamped and the heart is beating. This facilitates evacuation of atherosclerotic debris. Additional doses of cardioplegia solution are administered directly into each arteriotomy as it is made. Retrograde infusion of cardioplegia solution from the coronary sinus may be of advantage.[8]

3. Previously placed vein grafts are fully exposed and explored. If there is no visual evidence of atherosclerotic change and no palpable evidence of thickening, I do not replace them.

These special aspects of reoperation contribute to its distinctly higher mortality, which tends to increase with the time from the initial operation. Ten years or more following the initial operation, the risk of reoperation has been reported to be as high as 16%.[12]

COMBINED VALVULAR AND CORONARY BYPASS SURGERY

When valvular surgery is done in combination with coronary surgery, the coronary anastomoses are performed first. When valvular surgery is performed for aortic insufficiency, cardioplegia solution is administered by opening the ascending aorta and selectively cannulating the coronary ostia before doing the distal anastomoses. It is important to cannulate the right and left coronary ostia. The left ostium is posterior and readily visible. The right ostium is anterior. It is often poorly visualized until it is everted by pressure on the right ventricular outflow tract.

When ITA grafts are used, I have alternately clamped or not clamped the graft during the valvular surgery. One liter of cold crystalloid cardioplegia solution is administered every 10–15 minutes at the rate of 400 ml/min. Both clamping and not clamping ITA grafts have given very satisfactory results. This has also been true in relation to previous ITA grafts when reoperation has been required for valve replacement. Unlike reoperative coronary surgery, intermittent administration of cardioplegia solution through the coronary ostia maintains myocardial cooling.

COMBINED VENTRICULAR ANEURYSM RESECTION AND CORONARY BYPASS SURGERY

Ventricular aneurysms sometimes contain loose thrombus. I prefer to open the aneurysm, remove any loose clot, and repair the aneurysm prior to performing coronary surgery. The left ventricular vent cannula is disconnected from the venous gravity drainage line and attached to pump suction prior to incision into the aneurysm. Following aneurysm repair, the vent is again connected to the gravity venous line and coronary surgery is performed.

REFERENCES

1. Baird RJ, Dutka F, Okumari M: Surgical aspects of regional myocardial blood flow and myocardial pressure. *J Thorac Cardiovasc Surg* 69:17–29, 1975.

2. Akins CW: Noncardioplegic myocardial preservation for coronary revascularization. *J Thorac Cardiovasc Surg* 88:174–181, 1984.

3. Minale C, Nicol S, Zander M: Coronary endarterectomy: An old technique and new controversies. Treatment of End Stage Coronary Artery Disease. *J Adv Cardiol* 36(Suppl) 34–40, 1988.

4. Crosby IK, Wellons HA, Taylor GJ: Critical analysis of the preoperative and operative predictions of aorto-coronary bypass patency. *Ann Surg* 193:743–751, 1981.

5. Green GE, Som ML, Wolff WI: Experimental microvascular suture anastomosis. *Circulation* 33:I-199–I-203, 1966.

6. Green GE: Exposure of the circumflex coronary artery and its branches. *Surgery* 73:66–67, 1973.

7. Molina EJ, Galliani CA, Einzig S, et al: Physical and mechanical effects of cardioplegic injection on flow distribution and myocardial damage in hearts with normal coronary arteries. *J Thorac Cardiovasc Surg* 97:870–877, 1989.

8. Drinkwater DC, Laks H, Buckberg GD: A new simplified method of optimizing cardioplegic delivery without right heart isolation. *J Thorac Cardiovasc Surg* 100:56–64, 1990.

9. Shahian DM, Neptune WB, Ellis FH Jr: Intraaortic balloon pump mobidity: A comparative analysis of risk factors between percutaneous and surgical techniques. *Ann Thorac Surg* 36:644–651, 1983.

10. Verani MS, Mahmarian JJ, Cocanougher BB: Left ventricular function in patients with centrifugal left ventricular assist device. *ASAIO Trans* 35:544–547, 1989.

11. Nugent WC, Naislen EL, O'Connor GT: Pericardial flap prevents sternal wound complications. *Arch Surg* 123:636–639, 1986.

12. Salomon NW, Page SU, Bigelow JC: Reoperative coronary surgery. *J Thorac Cardiovasc Surg* 100:250–260, 1990.

CHAPTER **8**

Which Areas of Myocardium Should Be Revascularized With ITAs? Pedicle Grafts, Sequential Grafts, Free Grafts

GEORGE E. GREEN

Internal thoracic artery (ITA) grafts should be used for those areas of myocardium which are most important and most ischemic. Each ITA is capable of supplying one of the three major areas of myocardial perfusion—anterior [left anterior descending coronary artery (LAD) distribution], lateral (circumflex distribution), or posterior (right and/or circumflex distribution). Infrequently, I have used the ITAs to supply all three areas of distribution, as described by Sauvage et al.[1] (Fig. 8–1). Justification of such use is based on the capacity of the ITA for progressive dilatation and increase of flow.[2,3] The reservation about such use is possible ITA inadequacy.[4] My own reservations about using ITAs as the sole source of revascularization for all three major areas are two:

1. Basal normal myocardial blood flow is 80 ml/100 g/min,[5] but flow reserve is three- to fivefold.[6] Normal adult cardiac weight is 250–350 g. Flows from the transected ends of ITAs after mobilization average 138 ml/min.[7] Although ITA flow and size do increase with demand, the time required for such increase has not been defined.

2. A graft that allows a threefold increase in flow, the minimum required for normal coronary flow reserve, may not allow a six- or ninefold increase in flow—as would be necessary through the proximal left ITA (LITA) if it were the source of inflow for three major myocardial areas (Fig. 8–1). Because of these considerations, I usually use each ITA graft for one of the three major areas of myocardial perfusion.

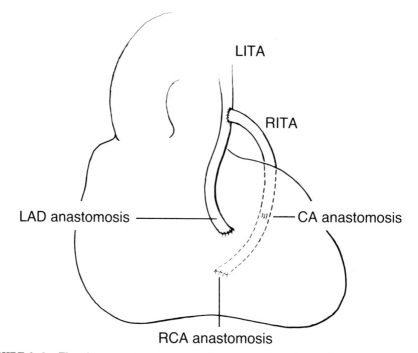

FIGURE 8–1 The three major areas can be reached with two ITAs if the right ITA is placed as a free graft arising from the left pedicle. In such instances, the flow capacity of the proximal portion of the LITA will have to be adequate for at least a ninefold increase. RCA = right coronary artery.

Pedicled ITA grafts should be used preferentially whenever possible because their long-term fate is more completely documented than that of free grafts. In most patients, the LITA pedicle graft can reach either the anterior or lateral aspects of the heart. If atherosclerosis is strictly localized, only one anastomosis will be required for each area of myocardium (Fig. 8–2A,B). Often atherosclerotic stenoses are diffuse. Minor areas of compromise (e.g., small diagonal branches of the LAD, small intermediate branches between the LAD and the circumflex artery, or small branches of the circumflex) can be safely ignored if good inflow into the major branches is achieved. For example, in the situation illustrated in Fig. 8–3, a sequential graft to the second diagonal branch of the LAD and the interventricular branch of the LAD has been done. The small first diagonal and intermediate branches have been ignored. Sequential anastomoses to the first and third lateral branches of the circumflex artery afford complete revascularization of the circumflex system.

Some areas of the right coronary distribution do not require specific surgical revascularization. Right ventricular branches of the right coronary artery are usually well collateralized from the LAD, have relatively little work demand, and therefore do not require specific revascularization. On the other hand, major areas of distribution of the right coronary artery to the left ventricle should not be ignored. Sequential anastomoses may be required, and to achieve sufficient length for these, a free graft may be needed. For example,

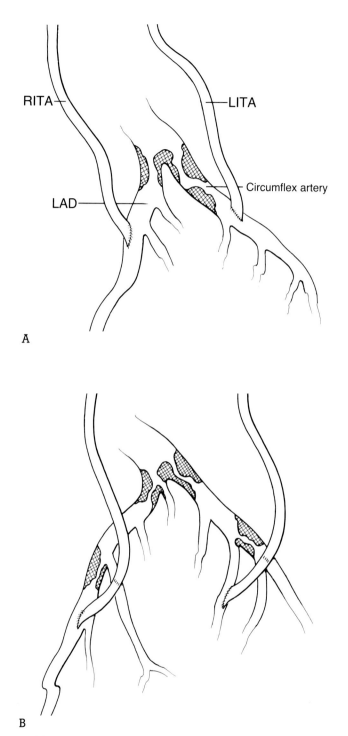

FIGURE 8-2 **A:** When atherosclerosis is localized, only one anastomosis is required for each area. **B:** When important subsidiary areas are compromised, sequential anastomoses are required.

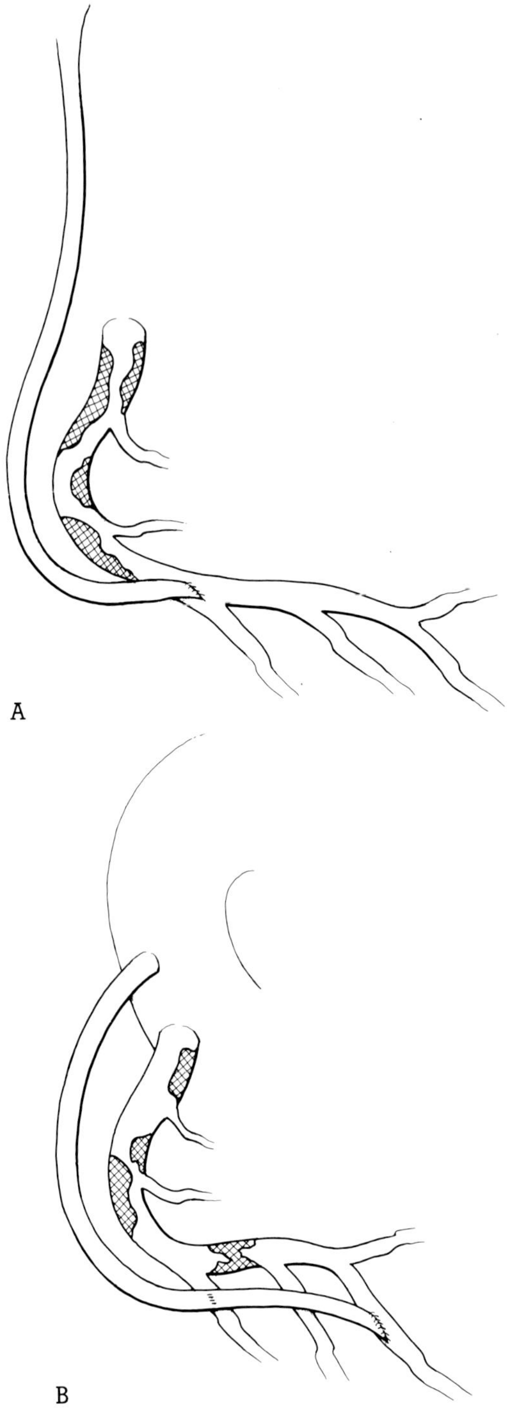

FIGURE 8–3 A: Pedicled RITA grafts usually reach the posterior descending artery (PDA). Stenoses of right ventricular branches of the right coronary artery (RCA) can usually be ignored. **B:** If a major posterior left ventricular (PLV) branch of the RCA is stenotic, sequential anastomosis is required. A free graft is usually needed to reach both the posterior descending (PDA) and posterior left ventricular branches of the RCA.

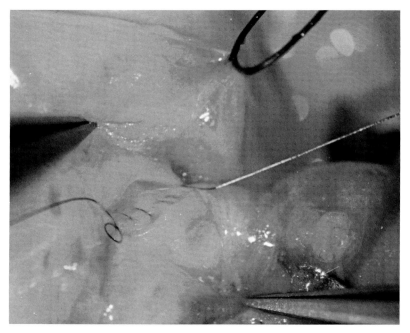

FIGURE 8-4 Parallel (axial) sequential anastomosis. Photographed through a microscope at 8×.

the posterior descending branch of the right coronary artery can usually be reached by a pedicled graft (Fig. 8–3A). A free graft is usually required to reach the posterior descending and posterior left ventricular branches of the right coronary artery (Fig. 8–3B). Special aspects of sequential and free grafts warrant comment.

SEQUENTIAL GRAFTS

Estimation of the length required from the origin of the graft to the sites of anastomoses is more demanding than with simple grafts. Inadequate length will cause disruption or late stricture. The length to the first (side-to-side) anastomosis is best judged when the heart is full. Even though selecting and marking sites for anastomoses is best done with the heart decompressed, the length of grafts is best determined by returning the heart to its normal position and allowing it to fill. Grafts to the diagonal and LAD branches can be laid on the anterior surface of the heart and appropriate spots on the pedicle marked with hemoclips. Lengths of the grafts to the lateral and posterior areas of the heart are best judged by returning the heart to its normal position, allowing it to fill, and marking the spots in the lateral or posterior pericardium that correspond to the epicardial site of projected anastomoses. The heart is then decompressed again and retracted. The graft is laid along the pericardium to the designated spots, which are marked on the pedicle with hemoclips. The proximal anastomosis of a sequential graft may be either parallel (axial—Fig. 8–4) or perpendicular (diamond—Fig. 8–5) to the coronary artery.

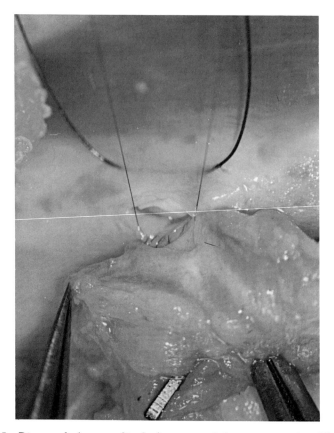

FIGURE 8–5 Diamond (perpendicular) sequential anastomosis. Photographed through a microscope at 8×.

The parallel anastomosis is easier to perform than the diamond anastomosis. Exposure is simpler, and arteriotomy length is not critical. However, the length of the pedicle between the proximal and distal anastomoses is critical because parallel anastomoses incur acute angulation of the graft if the length between the anastomoses is not ample (Fig. 8–6A,B). When arterial branches are divergent, as they usually are, long lengths of graft may be required to avoid acute angulation. The length required for the distal loop can be diminished by bringing the ITA perpendicular to the distal arteriotomy—T rather than parallel configuration (Fig. 8–7A–C). The problem of angulation of the distal loop can be eliminated by making the proximal anastomosis at a right angle to the coronary arteriotomy-diamond anastomosis. However, arteriotomy length is critical in diamond anastomoses. Too long an arteriotomy will cause "gull wing" deformity (Fig. 8–8A,B) of the ITA. Such deformity limits flow into both the side-to-side and end-to-side anastomoses. Arteriotomy length for diamond anastomoses should be limited to the diameter of the coronary artery. I prefer placing the diamond anastomosis to the smaller coronary branch. This permits an arteriotomy that will not incur gull wing deformity.

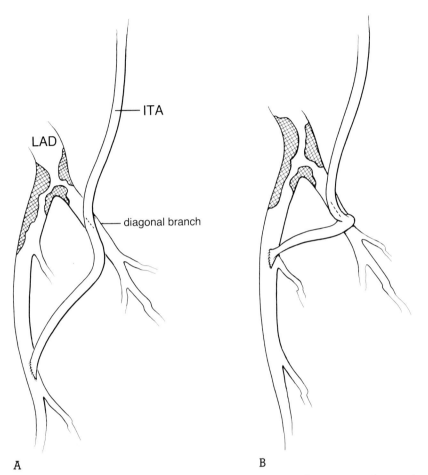

A   B

FIGURE 8–6 **A:** With a parallel configuration, sequential anastomosis requires a long loop to avoid kinking. **B:** With a parallel configuration, kinking of the graft at the proximal and distal anastomoses is caused by too short a loop.

A short arteriotomy demands precision. A diamond knife (Fig. 8–9) is extremely helpful. When properly cared for, its blade has unequaled sharpness. The area of the ITA chosen for the anastomosis should be thoroughly cleared of transverse thoracic fascia and muscle. Arteriotomy is most safely made with the artery distended. The adventitia of the graft is grasped with jewelers forceps (Fig. 8–10A–C). Countertraction is applied by the assistant. If the assistant is not familiar with microsurgery, a traction suture is placed in the adventitia. The adventitia is divided with several strokes of the diamond knife. The incision is deepened into the media. The bulging intima is divided. A microscissor (Fig. 8–11) is used if needed to extend the incision so that adventitia, media, and intima are coherent at the ends of the arteriotomy. High magnification is a great aid in guiding the hand for these maneuvers. Insufficient visualization, inappropriate traction, or an insufficiently sharp knife can result in disruption in the wall of the ITA. A disrupted area should

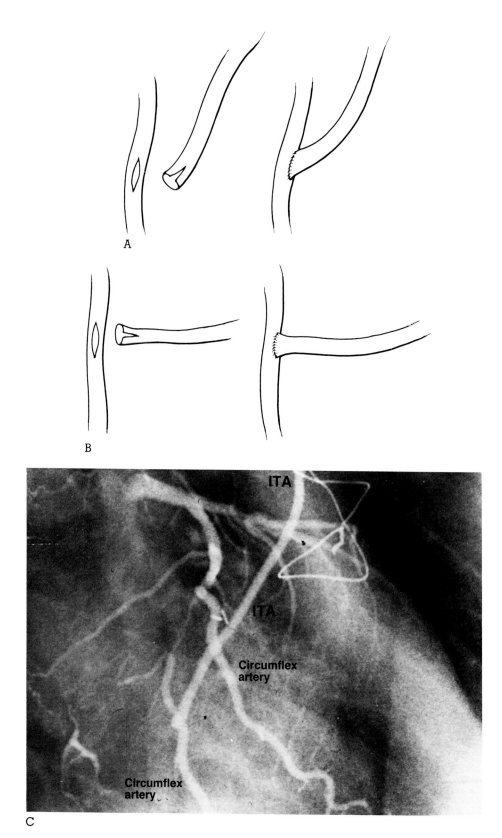

A

B

C

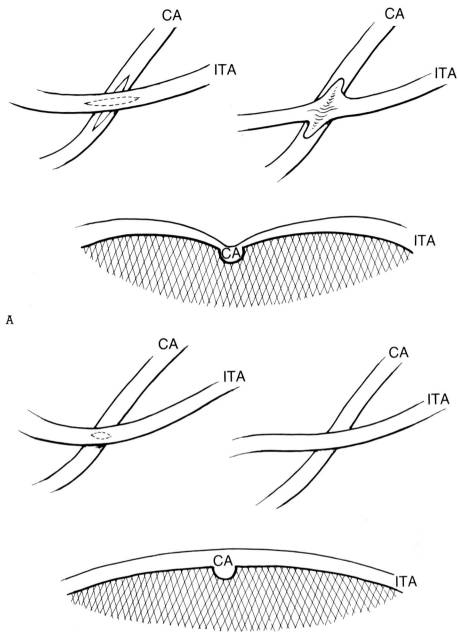

A

B

FIGURE 8–8 Gull wing deformity causes obstruction of flow into and out of a side-to-side anastomosis. **A:** The obstructive deformity is caused by an excessively long arteriotomy in the ITA and the graft. **B:** In contrast, arteriotomy no longer than the diameter of the ITA allows free flow. CA = coronary artery.

FIGURE 8–7 Length is saved and kinking at the anastomosis is avoided by making the anastomosis perpendicular to the arteriotomy. **A:** Parallel distal anastomosis requires more length than **B:** perpendicular "diamond" anastomosis. **C:** Postoperative angiogram of diamond anastomoses to two branches of the circumflex artery.

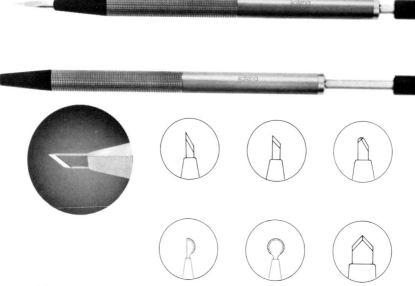

FIGURE 8-9 A diamond blade knife facilitates precise incision.

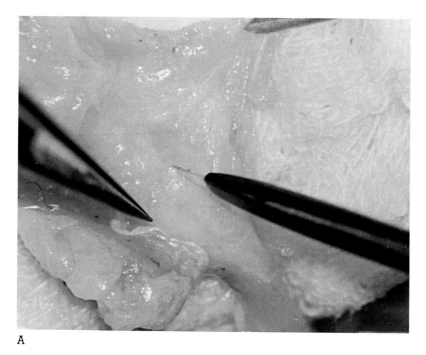

A

FIGURE 8-10 A: Arteriotomy begins with traction and countertraction on the adventitia. Photographed through a microscope at 8×.

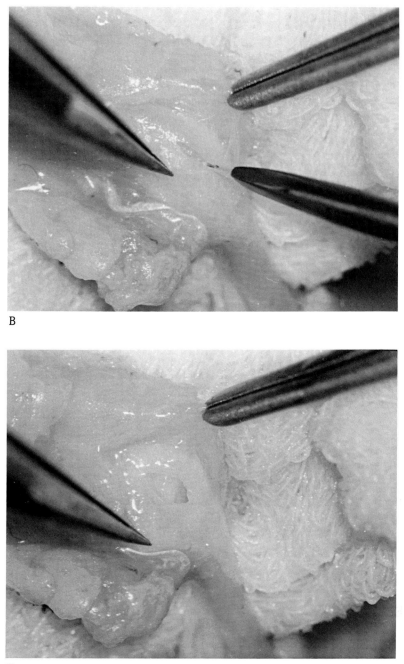

B

C

FIGURE 8–10 Continued B,C: After division of the adventitia, the bulging media and intima are divided. Photographed through a microscope at 8×.

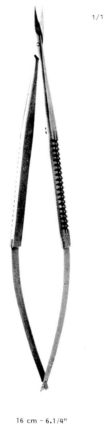

1/1

16 cm ~ 6.1/4"

FIGURE 8–11   Microscissor

not be used for anastomosis. Such an area should be excised. The residual normal segments are used as pedicled and free grafts (Fig. 8–12A–D).

Because of the technical demands of sequential anastomosis, two other modalities have been advocated for dealing with sequential coronary stenoses:

LASER ANGIOPLASTY

1. Laser angioplasty was first used in 1984.[8] No late patency data have been published. From personal knowledge, I am aware that angiographic studies of the first 11 argon laser angioplasties showed closure of the site of angioplasty 3 to 8 months after operation. Other lasers have been and are being evaluated (neodymium-YAG, carbon dioxide, eximer, dye tuned), but no late successes have been documented. At present, intraoperative laser angioplasty is not an alternative to sequential bypass.

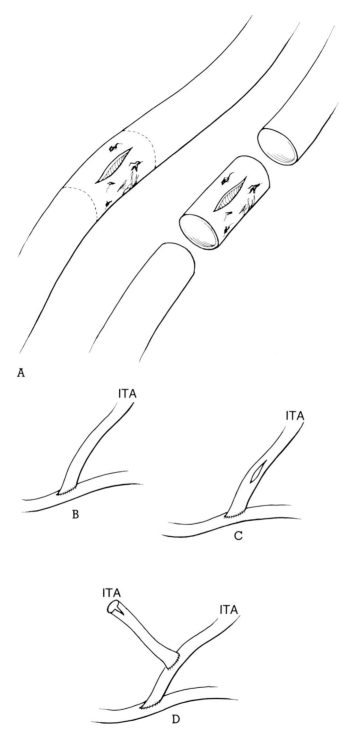

FIGURE 8–12 **A:** If the ITA is disrupted during arteriotomy, the area should be resected. **B:** The pedicled segment is used for end-to-side anastomosis. **C:** An arteriotomy is made in the pedicled graft. **D:** The free graft is joined to the pedicled graft.

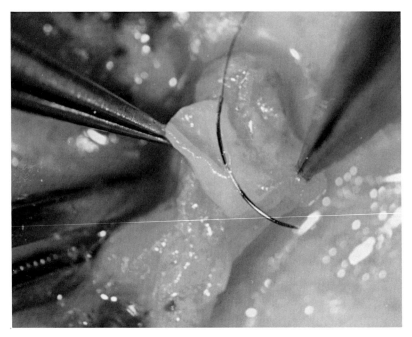

FIGURE 8–13 High magnification controls the depth of suture placement. Photographed through a microscope at 8×.

BALLOON ANGIOPLASTY

2. Intraoperative balloon angioplasty has been described as a convenient technique for dealing with sequential lesions.[9] This technique is less controlled than the angiographic technique from which it was derived. Approximately 5% of angiographically controlled balloon dilatations cause vessel disruption requiring surgical repair. Without angiographic control, disruption is more likely to occur and less likely to be recognized. Inadequate dilation and restenosis are more likely than problems with sequential anastomoses.

MAGNIFICATION AND SUTURE TECHNIQUES

Magnification and suture techniques are particularly pertinent to the side-to-side component of sequential anastomosis. Disruption of the wall of the ITA by arteriotomy, or too long an arteriotomy, can cause serious impairment of flow to both anastomoses. Excessive depth of suture placement can impair flow to both anastomoses. Depth of suture placement warrants comment. (Fig. 8–13). The length of hemostasis that can be achieved by any given suture is about equal to its depth. But as the depth of suture placement increases, the capacity of the artery for vasodilatation and flow reserve diminishes. Arteriotomy decompresses an artery, and its circumference becomes smaller. Excessive depth of suture placement is an important concern. The frequency of excessive depth of suture placement in ITA anastomoses is suggested by seven reports in an 18-month period which described percutaneous balloon dilatation for stenotic ITA-coronary anastomoses.[10] The hand requires visual guidance. Depth of the suture placement of 0.5 mm is required in coronary surgery.

Try the microscope you will like it

Try the microscope you will like it

Try the microscope you will like it

Try the microscope you will like it

Try the microscope you will like

Surgeons of many disciplines who work with structures comparable in size to coronary arteries routinely use the microscope—otologists, ophthalmologists, plastic surgeons, neurosurgeons, and orthopedic surgeons. In these disciplines, when the use of the instrument was initially advocated, the need for it was generally denied. After a critical number of surgeons—usually 20—tried it, its advantages were acknowledged and its use quickly became widespread. Surgeons in these disciplines now consider it fundamental to optimal technique. Learning to work with the operating microscope takes longer than learning to work with magnifying loupes—approximately 30 hours. This time is best spent in the laboratory, not in the clinical operating room. The effort is rewarded by greater surgical capacity and more comfortable working conditions. Magnifying loupes have considerable weight, and as the degree of magnification increases, so does the weight. Loupes require the surgeon's head and neck to be the focusing mechanism. It is necessary to work with a headlight, because the working distance is short and the surgeon's head blocks the illumination of the operating room light. By contrast, the operation microscope puts no weight on the surgeon's head and minimizes postural strain. Optics and illumination, as well as the focusing mechanism, are contained in the self-supporting microscope. Most important, with a wide range of magnification ($4\times-20\times$; Fig. 8–15A–E), the surgeon can work with confidence that blood vessel size will not limit surgical options.

Depth of suture placement is a critical factor in small blood vessel anastomosis. Increasing depth of suture placement enhances the possibility of stenosis or occlusion. Needle size determines the choice of suture because the needle is larger than the thread to which it swedged. Suture placement must be as deep as the diameter of the needle. The needle of a 6-0 suture has a diameter of 0.250 mm; the needle of a 7-0 suture has a diameter of 0.200 mm. To minimize the depth of suture placement, I use the smallest convenient needle. When vascular segments have diameters of 1.5 mm, I use the 8-0 suture, with a needle diameter 0.130 mm. When arterial segments are less than 1.5 mm, I prefer the 9-0 suture, with a needle diameter of 0.100 mm. [The size of coronary arteries is calibrated with probes of 0.25-mm gradation (Fig.

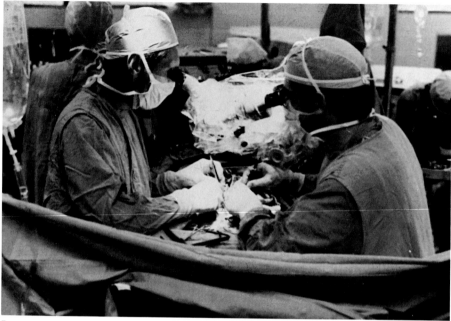

A

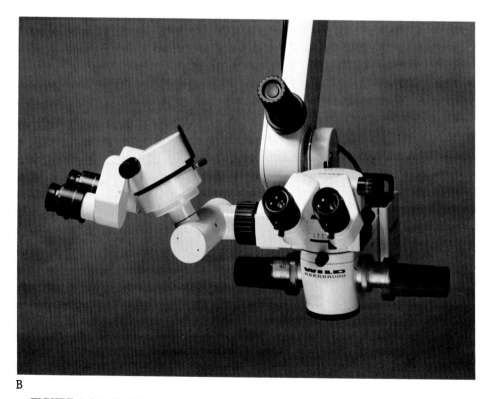

B

FIGURE 8–14 A: Microscope in use at surgery. **B:** Closeup of the microscope.

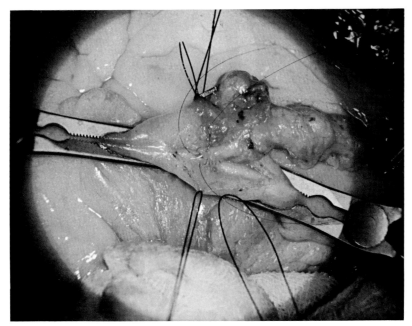

A

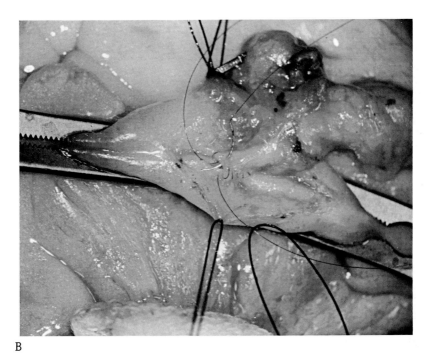

B

FIGURE 8–15 A–E: Nearly completed anastomosis photographed through a microscope at 4×, 6×, 8×, 12×, and 20×.

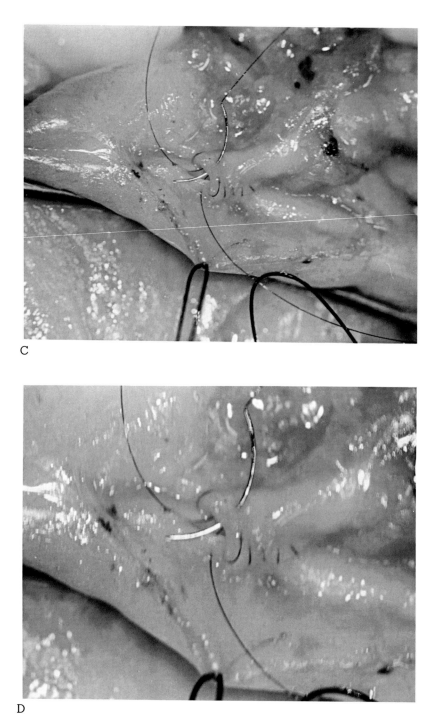

C

D

FIGURE 8–15 Continued

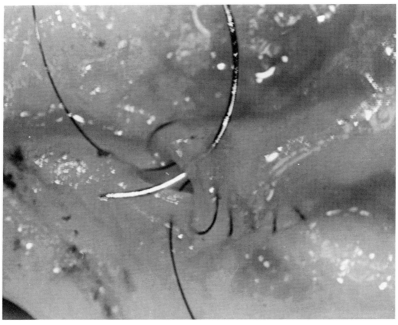

E

FIGURE 8–15 Continued

8–16A,B). The largest probe accommodated indicates the size of the artery.] Shallower depth of placement requires the use of more sutures. Usually 12 to 15 sutures are placed for each anastomosis. With 8× magnification the graft can be juxtaposed to the arteriotomy. Anastomosis time is reduced because both the graft and the arteriotomy are constantly in one field. Lesser degrees of magnification (optical loupes) require exposure techniques that preclude juxtaposition of the graft to the arteriotomy. Repeated change of field is time-consuming. Suturing time for a 12- to 15-bite anastomosis at a magnification of 8× is usually 7 minutes.

When a skilled assistant is working with the surgeon, traction on each successive stitch is made by the assistant as the surgeon makes countertraction with a jeweler's forceps on the arterial adventitia. An alternative technique, especially when not working with a skilled assistant, is to use a very short length of suture (approximately 6 cm). After the needle is grasped with the needle holder, traction is exerted by the suturing hand. A fine forceps held in the other hand grasps the appropriate adventitia. The needle is passed through the new site. When suturing is completed, the free ends are weighted by application of rubber-shod clamps. The needle is then avulsed from the suture. Using the needle as a hook, each loop of suture is drawn taut. This cannot be done without high magnification (Fig. 8–17A–K). Tying is done under visual control. Adjusting the tightness of the knot without visual control will sometimes break an 8-0 suture, will usually break a 9-0 suture, and can cause purse string stenosis (Fig. 8–18).

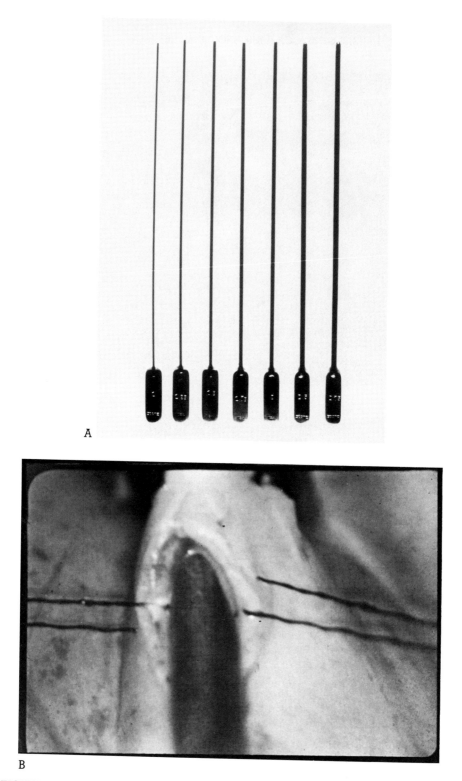

A

B

FIGURE 8–16 **A:** Probes of 0.25 mm calibration indicate the diameter of the artery. **B:** Probe in an artery. Photographed through a microscope at 8×.

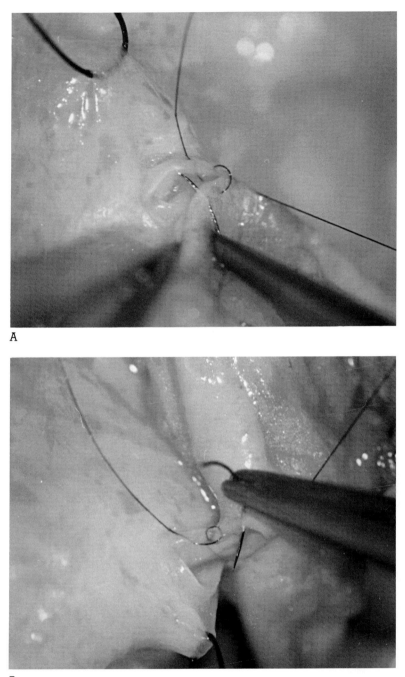

A

B

FIGURE 8–17 A–K: Side-to-side component of a sequential anastomosis. Continuous sutures have been laid in loosely. Each loop is secured by traction before the suture is tied. Photographed through a microscope at 8×.

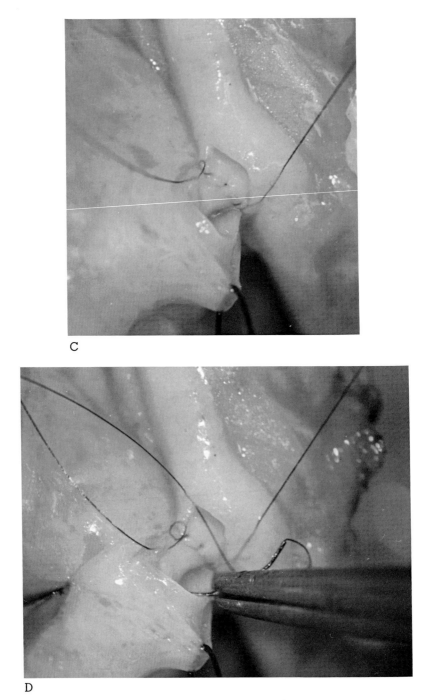

C

D

FIGURE 8–17 Continued

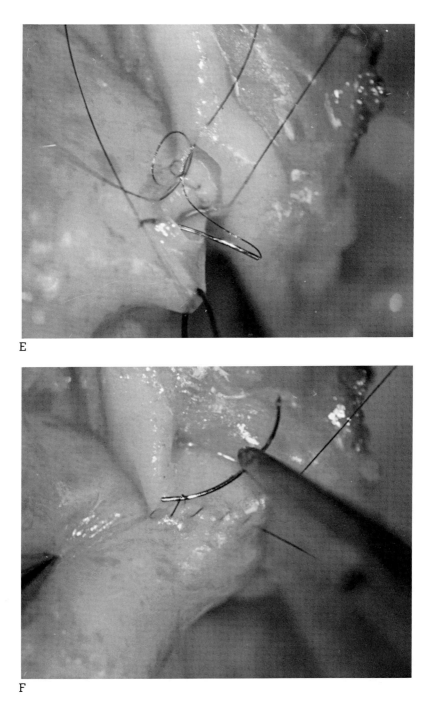

E

F

FIGURE 8–17 Continued

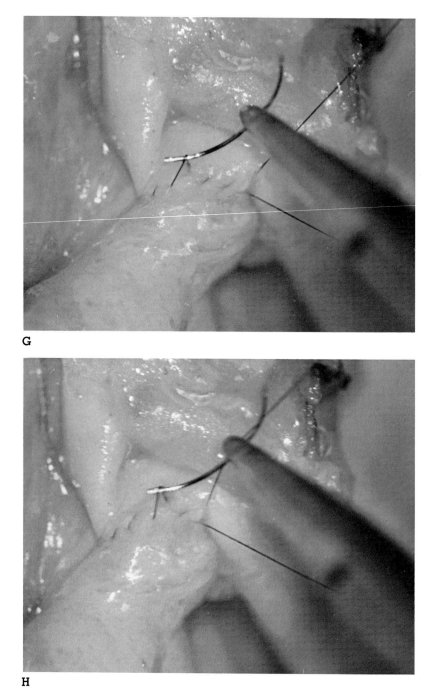

G

H

FIGURE 8–17 Continued

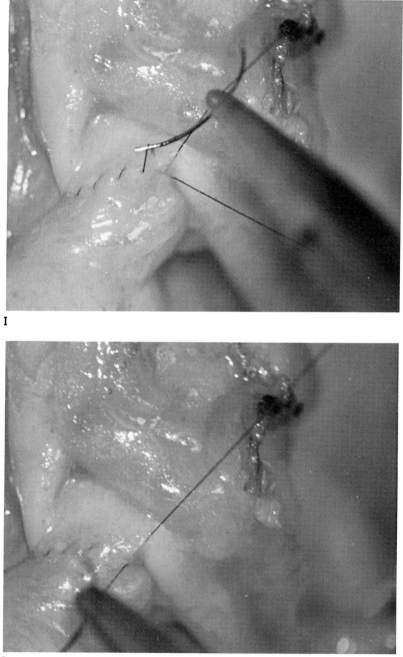

I

J

FIGURE 8–17 Continued

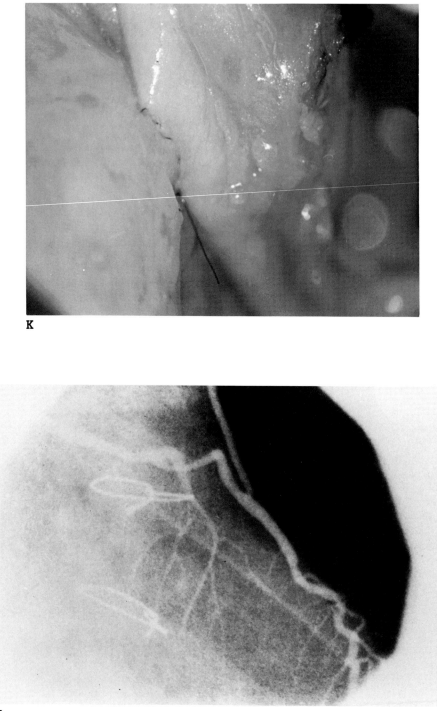

K

A

FIGURE 8–18   **A–C:** Examples of purse string stenoses. The anastomoses were made with 7-0 Prolene and tied too tightly.

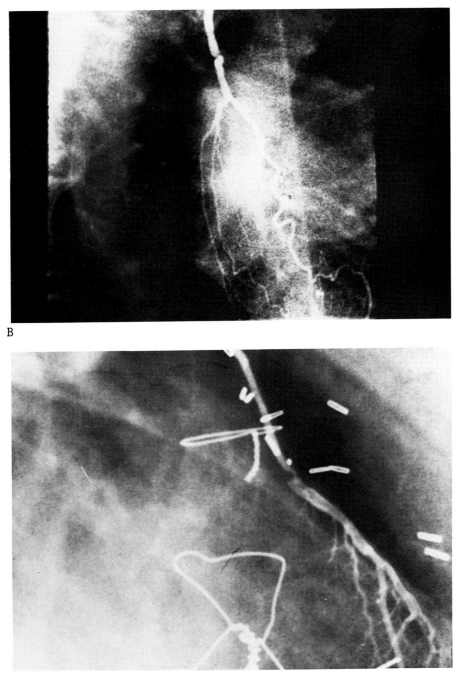

B

C

FIGURE 8–18 Continued

SHORT ITA SEGMENTS AS FREE GRAFTS

Using a short terminal segment of the pedicled ITA as a free graft is a way to salvage a damaged ITA pedicle and to make a pedicled graft more versatile.

If an ITA pedicle is damaged by mobilization or arteriotomy (for side-to-side anastomosis), the damaged area should not be included as part of the pedicled graft. After resection of the damaged area, the good segments can be used as pedicled and/or free grafts.

Short free segments of ITA are useful as grafts to high diagonal branches of the LAD for two reasons:

1. Exposure of high diagonal branches requires the heart to be drawn so far forward that a very long length of a LITA pedicle is required to reach the coronary segment. After side-to-side anastomosis, there may be insufficient length or diameter for the important intraventricular branch.

2. Side-to-side anastomoses are more difficult than end-to-side anastomoses. The ITA pedicle is more readily manipulated than an inaccessible coronary segment. When exposure is difficult, it is easier to perform two end-to-side anastomoses than one side-to-side anastomosis (see Fig. 8–18).

LONG ITA SEGMENTS AS FREE GRAFTS FROM THE AORTA

These were first described by Loop et al. 1973.[11] They were used in situations in which the ITA could not reach the coronary area as a pedicled graft. When the free graft was first introduced, I doubted its value. I had assumed that the high patency of ITA grafts was due to their pedicled nature. Unlike saphenous vein grafts, they carried their vasa vasorum intact and therefore were not subject to the ischemic damage that always affected saphenous vein grafts, sometimes causing early thrombosis and sometimes fibrotic stricture or occlusion.[12]

By 1982, Singh and Sosa had collated angiographic data on patients who had had vein grafts in addition to ITA grafts and were being restudied for recurrent angina (mean interval of 7 years after operation). Ninety-two percent of ITA grafts appeared perfect. Fifty percent of saphenous grafts, in contrast, were occluded, and atherosclerotic deformities were demonstrated in half of the others. Whereas early thrombosis and intimal fibrosis had affected only 10 to 20% of grafts, late atherosclerosis was affecting the majority of grafts.[13] I speculated that ITA pedicle grafts might be spared atherosclerosis because the integrity of their vasa maintained the integrity of the arterial wall. In 1985 I learned from Loop that he had reviewed late angiograms of 25 free ITA grafts Fig. 8–19 (performed more than 5 years after operation) and had seen no evidence of atherosclerotic or fibrotic change in these grafts. Reflecting on Loop's observations, I thought free ITA grafts might carry their

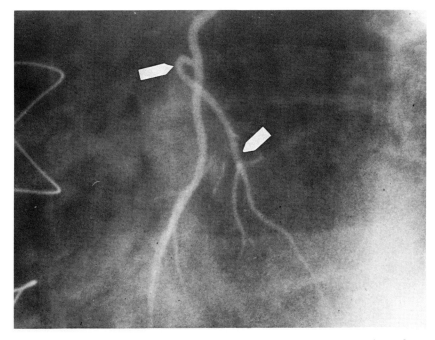

FIGURE 8–19 Postoperative angiogram of a free ITA segment (arrow) used instead of sequential anastomosis for revascularization of the LAD and its diagonal branch.

own vasa with them. Intercostal branches were conspicuous at regular intervals along the ITA. Vasa might arise from them. Injection of barium gel into postmortem specimens confirmed that the vasa of the ITA did in fact fill from the intercostal branches (Fig. 8–20A,B). In contrast, injection of radial artery segments (from just above the wrist to just below the elbow) showed no evidence of opacification of the vasa vasorum (Fig. 8–21A,B). Radial artery grafts were known to be uniformly subject to fibrotic stricture.[14,15] Loop's observations on the absence of late atherosclerosis or fibrosis in free ITA grafts, and my observations that ITA grafts retained their vasa and that these were probably functional as soon as the grafts were anastomosed to the aorta, encouraged me to extend their use. This encouragement was reinforced strongly by Sims' discovery and emphasis of the unique anatomy of the internal elastic lamina of the ITA.[16,17]

Although Loop found no late changes in the body of free ITA grafts, he emphasized that stricture of the proximal anastomosis was a serious problem. I believed then and still believe that anastomotic stricture is a technical problem that can be eliminated by appropriate surgical technique. Strictures caused by suturing occur as soon as the anastomosis is completed. By performing proximal anastomosis first and measuring the flow from the distal end of the graft, suture strictures can be discovered.

The technical problem of securely suturing the thin-walled ITA to the thick-walled aorta seemed formidable, but it was solved by the same high-magnification technique used for distal anastomoses. A 7-0 Prolene suture

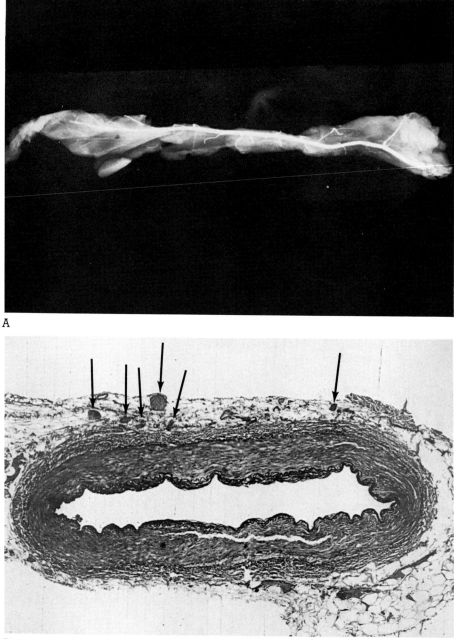

A

B

FIGURE 8–20   A: Barium gel injection of an isolated ITA specimen fills many intercostal branches. **B:** Microscopy shows barium gel in the vasa (arrows) of the adventitia of the ITA.

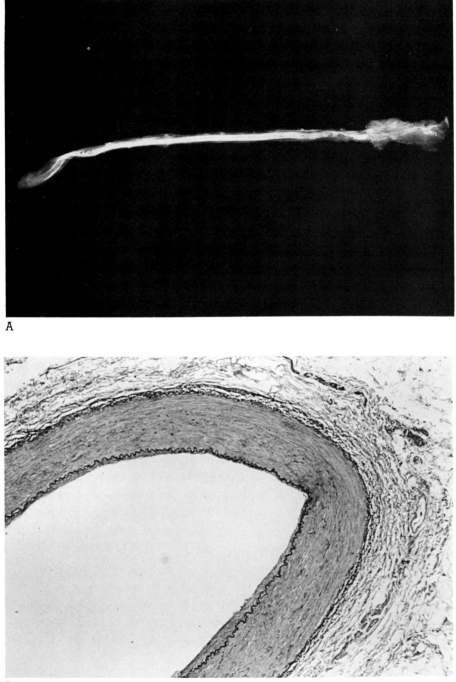

A

B

FIGURE 8–21 A: Barium gel injection of an isolated radial artery specimen shows no branches. **B:** Microscopy confirms the absence of barium gel in the vasa of the adventitia of the radial artery.

was substituted for the 8-0 Prolene suture in order to have a needle long enough to pass through the aortic wall. Separate passage of the needle through the ITA and the aorta is necessary. The torque required to pass the needle through both the ITA and the aorta is likely to tear the ITA. Sutures should be placed very close to the aortotomy so that the depth of suture placement into the ITA can be minimized. Deep bites cause distortion and stricture formation.

Anastomosis of the ITA to the aorta is performed with a partial occlusion clamp on the aorta. Arterial pressure should be kept low—a mean of 50 mm—to facilitate manipulation of the aorta. A small aortotomy is made using high magnification as a control. I prefer to make a V incision with a No. 11 blade. An ordinary rongeur is used to bite through the thick aortic media and intima. Adventitia is transected with a scissor (Fig. 8–22A–D). A longitudinal slit is made in the proximal segment of the ITA so that its total circumference matches that of the aortotomy. A continuous suture is used. This requires 20–25 suture bites. As with distal anastomoses, after all sutures have been placed, each loop is tightened and then the knot is tied with visual control (Fig. 8–23A–E). The anastomosis takes 15 minutes to complete. This is twice as long as distal anastomoses because there are twice as many suture bites, and because it is necessary to pass the needle separately through the ITA and the aorta. When the aortic clamp is released, the graft should appear distinctly larger than before anastomosis and flow from the distal end and should be copious—usually more than 200 ml/min. Flow should not be affected by swinging the graft through a wide arc. A positional nature of flow indicates suture stricture. Additional anastomotic sutures are rarely necessary. If additional sutures are placed, flow must be checked again following placement and adequacy of the anastomosis judged.

When the aorta is dramatically thickened, a small aortotomy is not feasible. If the aortotomy is so large that the ITA does not readily drape over it, a vein patch should be sutured to the aortotomy. ITA anastomosis can then be made through an incision in the vein patch.[18] Alternatively, the ITA can be sutured to an incision in the aortic hood of a saphenous vein graft. Although atherosclerosis rarely develops in the hood of saphenous vein grafts, I have seen it and prefer anastomosis directly to the aorta when feasible.

GRAFTS TO SEPTAL BRANCHES

Consideration of the possible need for revascularization of septal branches is warranted. It is known that critical ischemia to the septal area of the bundle of His can be lethal.[19] What constitutes critical ischemia is not clearly established. Over the course of 22 years, I have performed about 5,000 coronary bypass operations, with about 50 mortalities. I believe some of these mortalities were due to septal ischemia. These were unusual situations in which there was no existing or potential collateral flow to a stenotic major septal branch. I believe that septal branches 2 mm in diameter or more that are severely stenotic and will not be collateralized by grafts to either LAD or posterior descending artery (PDA) (due to diffuseness of disease) should be considered for direct revascularization. I believe that bypass is preferable to the techni-

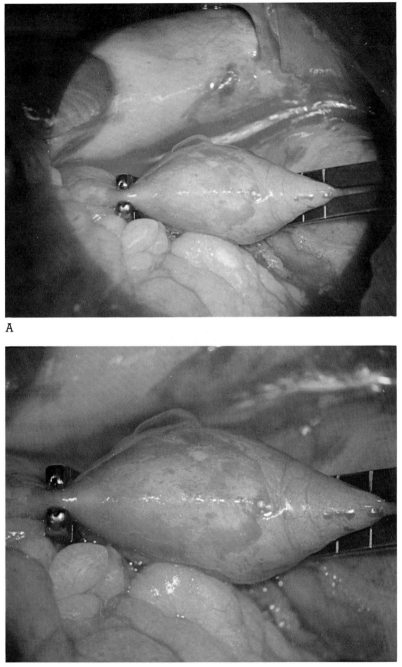

A

B

FIGURE 8–22 A–D: Partial occlusion clamp on the aorta for anastomosis of the ITA. Photographed through a microscope at 4×, 6×, and 8×.

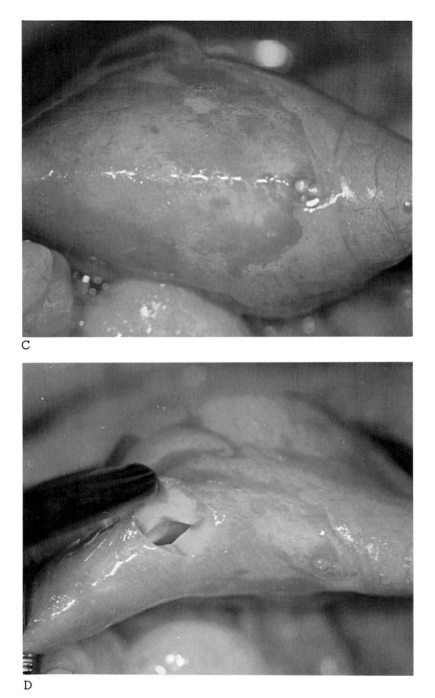

FIGURE 8–22 Continued

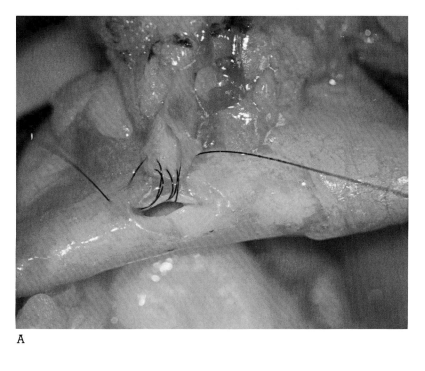

A

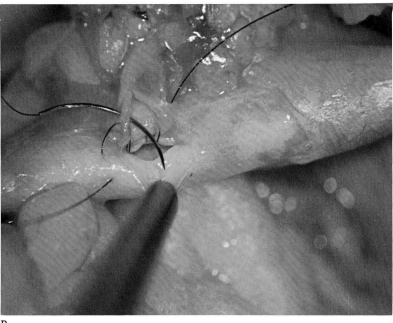

B

FIGURE 8–23 A–E: Suturing and adjusting the tension of sutures for an ITA graft to the aorta. Photographed through a microscope at 8×.

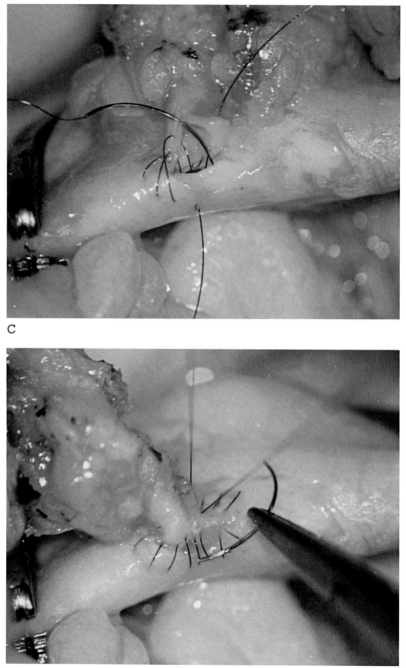

C

D

FIGURE 8–23 Continued

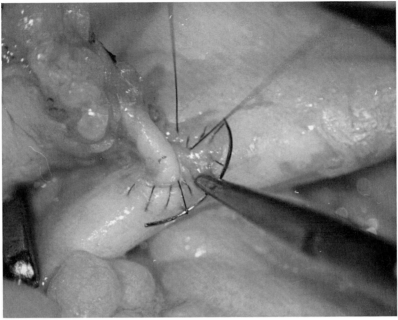

E

FIGURE 8–23 Continued

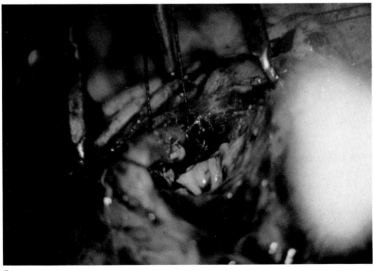

A

FIGURE 8–24   A: The first septal branch is detached from the LAD for anastomosis. Photographed through a microscope at 8×. (Figures 8–24 A–C appear in color after chapter 8.)

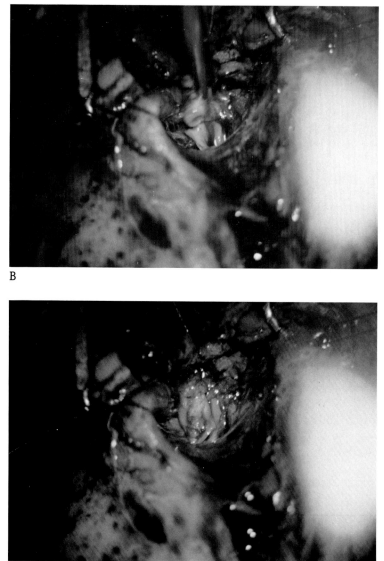

B

C

FIGURE 8–24 Continued   B,C: The ITA is sutured to the first septal branch. Photographed through a microscope at 8×.

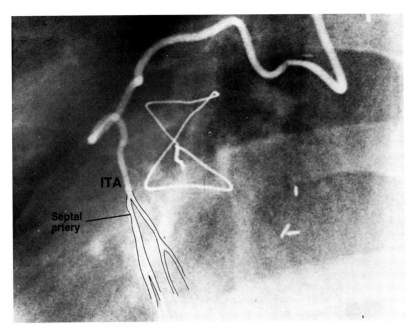

FIGURE 8–25 Angiogram of an ITA graft to the first septal artery 8 months after operation.

cally simpler procedure of endarterectomy. Bypass to major septal branches of the LAD requires traction on the trunk of the LAD to bring the septal branch as far out of the myocardium as is feasible. These intramyocardial portions of the septal branches are exceedingly thin-walled. High magnification is required for mobilization, arteriotomy, and anastomosis (Figs. 8–24, 8–25).

REFERENCES

1. Sauvage LR, Wu HD, Kowalsky TE, et al: Healing basis and surgical techniques for complete revascularization of the left ventricle using only the internal mammary arteries. *Ann Thorac Surg* 42:449–465, 1986.
2. Singh RN, Sosa JA: Internal mammary artery: A "live conduit" for coronary bypass. *J Thorac Cardiovasc Surg* 87:936–938, 1984.
3. Lee CN, Orszulak TA, Kaye MP: Flow capacity of the canine internal mammary artery. *J Thorac Cardiovasc Surg* 91:405–410, 1986.
4. Jones EL, Lattouf OM, Weintraub WS: Catastrophic consequences of internal mammary artery hypoperfusion. *J Thorac Cardiovasc Surg* 98:902–907, 1989.
5. Schmidt DH, Ray G: *Coronary Artery Surgery: Application of New Technologies.* Chicago, Year Book Medical Publishers, 1983, p 59.
6. Wilson RF, White CW: Intracoronary papaverine: An ideal coronary vasodilator for studies of the coronary circulation in conscious humans. *Circulation* 73:444–451, 1986.

7. Green GE: Rate of blood flow from the internal mammary artery. *Surgery* 70:809–813, 1971.

8. Choy DSJ, Stertzer SH, Myler RK: Human laser coronary recanalization. *Clin Cardiol* 7:377–381, 1984.

9. Urschcel HC, Razzuk MA, Miller E: Operative transluminal balloon angioplasty. *J Thorac Cardiovasc Surg* 99:581–589, 1990.

10. Green GE: Expanded role of the internal mammary artery. *Current Opinion Cardiol* 2:987–989, 1987.

11. Loop FD, Spampinato N, Cheanvechai C: The free internal mammary artery bypass graft: Use of the IMA in the aorta-to-coronary position. *Ann Thorac Surg* 15:50–55, 1973.

12. Campeau L, Lesperance J, Bourassa MG: Natural history of saphenous vein aorto-coronary bypass grafts. *Mod Concepts Cardiovasc Dis* 53:59–63, 1984.

13. Singh RN, Sosa JA, Green GE: Long term fate of the internal mammary artery and saphenous vein grafts. *J Thorac Cardiovasc Surg* 86:359–363, 1983.

14. Curtis JJ, Stoney WS, Alfred WCJ: Internal hyperplasia: A cause of radial artery aorto-coronary bypass graft failure. *Ann Thorac Surg* 20:628–635, 1975.

15. Chiu C: Why do radial artery grafts fail? A reappraisal. *Ann Thorac Surg* 22:520–523, 1976.

16. Sims FH: Discontinuities in the internal elastic lamina: A comparison of coronary and internal mammary arteries. *Artery* 13:127–143, 1985.

17. Sims FH, Gavin JB, Vanderwee MA: The intima of human coronary arteries. *Am Heart J* 118:32–38, 1989.

18. Schimert G, Vidne BA, Lee AB Jr: Free internal mammary artery graft: An improved surgical technique. *Ann Thorac Surg* 19:474–477, 1975.

19. James TN, Riddick L: Sudden death due to isolated acute infarction of its bundle. *J Am Coll Cardiol* 15:1183–1187, 1980.

COLOR PLATES

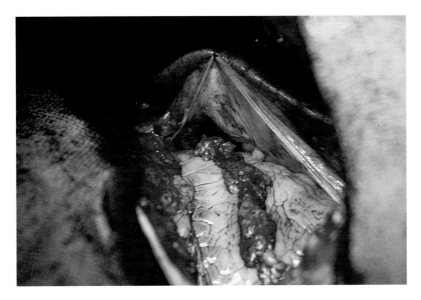

PLATE 1   The left ITA is brought through the pleuropericardial fold near the phrenic nerve.

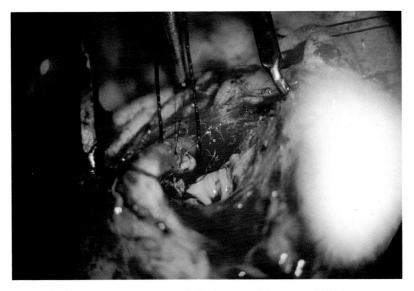

PLATE 2   The first septal branch is detached from the LAD for anastomosis. Photographed through a microscope at 8×.

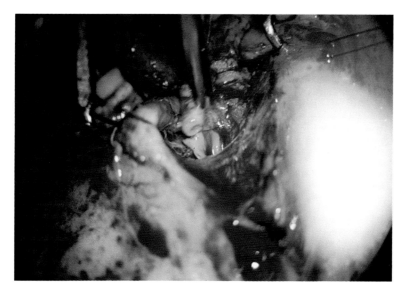

PLATE 3

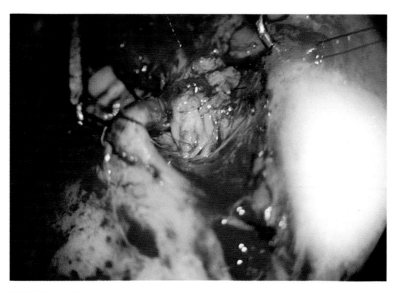

PLATE 4 The ITA is sutured to the first septal branch. Photographed through a microscope at 8×.

CHAPTER 9

The Internal Thoracic Artery in Pediatric Cardiac Surgery

GEORGE E. GREEN

ANOMALOUS ORIGIN OF THE LEFT CORONARY ARTERY

Anomalous origin of the left coronary artery from the pulmonary artery was the first pediatric coronary condition to receive cardiac surgical attention. In utero, because of wide patency of the ductus arteriosus, the anomalous left coronary artery is perfused by partially oxygenated blood. Myocardial work and oxygen demand are low in utero but rise abruptly at birth. As the ductus arteriosus closes, pulmonary artery resistance and pressure diminish. The myocardium, previously perfused by the anomalous left coronary artery, now becomes dependent upon collateral circulation. But as the pulmonary artery pressure of the newborn continues to drop, the direction of flow in the anomalous artery reverses. Blood drains from the left coronary artery into the pulmonary artery, causing more impairment of myocardial perfusion. Initial surgical attention was directed to interrupting the coronary-pulmonary steal. The anomalous coronary artery was ligated at its origin.[1] Subsequently, corrective measures were added. A Dacron graft from the ascending aorta was the first operation used to restore antegrade arterial flow.[2] Later, autogenous vein grafts[3] and then subclavian artery–coronary artery anastomoses were used.[4] Because of the preferential long-term patency of internal thoracic artery (ITA) grafts, because of the limited length of the subclavian artery, and because there are drawbacks to interruption of the subclavian artery, it is logical that ITA anastomosis should be used. To date, this has been used only to correct atresia of the left coronary artery.[5]

KAWASAKI DISEASE

Kawasaki's disease, an acute febrile illness of infants and young children characterized by florid inflammatory lesions of the skin, mucous membranes, and lymph nodes, can affect coronary arteries.[6] The initial change, vasculitis, is followed by aneurysmal dilatation. Late stricture formation or thrombosis can ensue. Surgical relief of the myocardial ischemia caused by Kawasaki's disease was first attempted with saphenous vein grafts. Late closure of these grafts was the rule. Pedicled ITA grafts were evaluated, and high patency was observed. Growth in the length as well as the diameter of the graft was documented.[7]

CORRECTIONS OF COARCTATIONS AND CREATION OF SHUNTS

The ITA has been used to extend the length of the subclavian artery for subclavian flap repairs of aortic coarctation and for Blalock systemic-pulmonary shunts. Because of its remarkable growth capacity, the ITA has been used successfully as a pedicled graft (without interrupting the subclavian artery) for systemic-pulmonary shunts.[8,9] More recently, this same capacity prompted its use to correct problems encountered in arterial switch operations. When the length of the left or right coronary artery is inadequate for ostial translocation, catastrophic myocardial ischemia can ensue. This has been successfully alleviated by ITA anastomosis to the affected coronary artery.[10,11]

REFERENCES

1. Sabiston DC, Orme SK: Congenital origin of the left coronary artery from the pulmonary artery. *J Thorac Cardiovasc Surg* 9:543, 1968.
2. Cooley DA, Hallman GL, Bloodwell RD: Definitive surgical treatment of anomalous origin of left coronary artery from pulmonary artery. *J Thorac Cardiovasc Surg* 52:798–808, 1966.
3. El Said GM, Ruzyllo W, William RL: Early and late results of saphenous vein for anomalous origin of left coronary artery from the pulmonary artery. *Circulation* 47, 48(pt 2):III-2–III-9, 1973.
4. Meyer BW, Slefanik D, Stiles QR: A method of definitive surgical treatment of anomalous origin of left coronary artery. *J Thorac Cardiovasc Surg* 56:104–107, 1968.
5. Fortune RL, Baron PJ, Fitzgerald JW: Atresia of the left main coronary artery: Repair with left internal mammary artery bypass. *J Thorac Cardiovasc Surg* 94:150–151, 1987.
6. Fauci AS: *Cecil Textbook of Medicine*. Philadelphia, WB Saunders, 1985, p 1940.
7. Kitamura S, Kawachi K, Seki T: Bilateral internal mammary artery grafts for coronary artery bypass operations in children. *J Thorac Cardiovasc Surg* 99:708–715, 1990.

8. Cobanoglu A, Abbruzzes P, Braumer D: Therapeutic considerations in congenital absence of the right pulmonary artery. Use of internal mammary artery as a preparatory shunt. *J Thorac Cardiovasc Surg* 25:241, 1984.

9. Sievers H, Lange P, Heintsen P: Internal mammary artery as a palliative systemic—pulmonary shunt. *J Thorac Cardiovasc Surg* 33:51, 1984.

10. Ebels T, Meuzelaar K, Gallandat Huet RCG: Neonatal arterial switch operation complicated by intramural left coronary artery and treated by left internal mammary artery bypass graft. *J Thorac Cardiovasc Surg* 97:473–475, 1989.

11. Rheuban KS, Kron IL, Bulatovic A: Internal mammary artery bypass after the arterial switch operation. *Ann Thorac Surg* 50:125–126, 1990.

CHAPTER **10**

Intraoperative and Postoperative Blood Loss: Reoperation for Bleeding

GEORGE E. GREEN

Blood loss with coronary bypass surgery is related to so many factors that comparison of groups of patients operated on in different time periods or in different institutions is not meaningful. Some of the factors determining blood loss are:

Preoperative medication
Anesthetic technique
Surgical technique
Mode of heart-lung bypass
Blood conservation program

In my practice, since 1985, 90% of patients undergoing coronary bypass surgery have had multiple internal thoracic artery (ITA) anastomoses. This has involved the use of both ITAs in more than 80% of patients. The number of anastomoses per patient has averaged 3.5. Two-thirds of all anastomoses have been constructed from ITAs. Blood transfusion has been required in half of the patients operated on. Average administration of blood has been 2 units of packed cells per patient. Surgical reexploration has been needed in 1%.[1,2] Aspects that warrant comment will now be discussed.

PREOPERATIVE MEDICATION

Fibrinolytic agents—tissue-type plasminogen activator (tPA), streptokinase (SK), and urokinase (UKN)—are administered to a significant number of pa-

186

tients with acute myocardial ischemia. When severe ischemia persists despite administration of these agents, urgent surgical intervention may be necessary. Although the half-life of the activating agent is short—less than 1 hour—its effects are prolonged. Depletion of fibrinogen, prothrombin, and factors V, VII, and XII can be documented for 12 hours following administration. Moreover, there is persistence of fibrin split products which have anticoagulant activity. Urgent surgical intervention in patients who have been receiving fibrinolytic agents will surely be complicated by excessive bleeding. Bleeding can be diminished by administering several agents. Aminocaproic acid (10 g) is given after heparinization but before initiating heart-lung bypass. Desmopressin (0.3 mg/kg) should be administered 15 minutes before terminating heart-lung bypass. Cryoprecipitate (12 units) and blood platelets are given soon after protamine. Aminocaproic acid prevents further conversion of plasminogen to plasmin. In high doses it partially blocks the action of the plasmin. Aprotinin (Trasylol) is claimed to be more effective but is not yet available for use in the United States. Desmopressin enhances platelet activity. It may return dysfunctional platelets (made so by heparin and the heart-lung machine) toward normal. Cryoprecipitate restores coagulation factors.

Aspirin is notorious for its capacity to impair blood platelet function for the duration of the life of the blood platelet—10 days. A completely normal platelet population requires cessation of aspirin therapy 10 days before operation. I advocate this for all stable patients. Patients who are so unstable that operation cannot be safely deferred are operated on urgently, but with the awareness that impaired hemostasis may be unusually severe. Patients who have stopped taking aspirin well in advance of surgery have a normal preoperative bleeding time. Surprisingly, many patients who have taken aspirin up to the time of operation have also had normal preoperative bleeding times. Such patients have not required platelet transfusion or had excessive blood loss. However, they have received aminocaproic acid (10 g) immediately after heparinization and desmopressin (0.300 µg/kg) prior to discontinuing heart-lung bypass. Patients who have taken aspirin up to the time of surgery and have elevated bleeding times usually require platelet transfusions because of obvious coagulopathy—i.e., no evidence of blood clot after administration of protamine. Despite administration of aminocaproic acid, desmopressin, and platelets, these patients have also required multiple blood transfusions.

Drugs other than aspirin can impair platelet function. Some can be discontinued before surgery, such as clofibrate, sulfinpyrazone, and tricyclic antidepressants. Others cannot be avoided, including penicillin and related antibiotics, propranalol, and related beta blockers.

ANESTHETIC TECHNIQUE

Blood loss during mobilization of ITA grafts is minimized by keeping systolic blood pressure no higher than 100 mm Hg. However, prior to chest closure, while hemostasis is being assayed and ensured, it is extremely important that blood pressure be raised above 100 mm Hg. During the initial hours after operation, as anesthesia wears off, blood pressure tends to rise. For several hours after operation, blood pressure should not be allowed to rise above the level at which the chest wall was scrutinized. The alpha-blocking action of chlorpromazine is helpful in this early postoperative phase.

SURGICAL TECHNIQUE

Mobilization of ITA grafts was discussed in Chapter 6, but some aspects warrant reemphasis. High-intensity cautery should be avoided because it causes excessive tissue damage, but also because it confers poor hemostasis. Too high an intensity disrupts vascular structures before hemostasis is achieved. In the presence of a bleeding diathesis, ligature or hemoclip control of bleeding is preferable to cautery. All coronary anastomoses should be scrutinized for bleeding during heart-lung bypass at a mean pressure of 100 mm. Gentle traction on the grafts is helpful in exposing any jet of bleeding from the anastomosis. Such bleeding should be controlled by suture. Oozing will generally cease with restoration of normal coagulation, but a jet of blood must be controlled surgically.

It is desirable to close the pleuropericardial folds over the heart and grafts. Ample posterior pericardial drainage by incision through the posterior pleuropericardial fold will minimize the occurrence of cardiac tamponade or compression.

MODE OF HEART-LUNG BYPASS

All currently available oxygenators diminish the platelet population by causing aggregation. The residual platelets manifest degranulation and an impaired capacity for agglutination. No statistically significant data differentiate the behavior of bubble oxygenators from that of membrane oxygenators in regard to platelet dysfunction. Little has been published concerning the effects of different types of oxygenators on factors in the coagulation cascade. Nevertheless, it is my impression that bubble oxygenators have more potential for causing blood damage than membrane oxygenators. The direct contact of oxygen with blood is harmful. Increasing intensity of contact is increasingly harmful. In former years, it was possible to diminish the contact of blood with oxygen in bubble oxygenators by reducing oxygen flow until arterial oxygen tension was in the range of 90–100 mm Hg. However, the current design of bubble oxygenators provides such extensive exposure of blood to oxygen that oxygen flow cannot be reduced to a level affording less oxygen exposure (arterial oxygen saturation = 90%) without incurring excessive accumulation of carbon dioxide. I therefore have used the silicon sheet membrane oxygenator since 1987.

Strong suction causes turbulent mixing of blood and air, which is damaging to platelets and blood cells. Prolonged, forceful suction should be avoided. Connecting the ventricular vent to the gravity venous line is helpful in this regard.

BLOOD CONSERVATION PROGRAM

Following heart-lung bypass, all blood in the heart-lung machine should be reinfused to the patient, either by direct infusion before decannulation or later by a blood transfusion bag.

Because of the defibrinating capacity of the pleural and pericardial membranes, most of the blood shed into the chest during and after operation can be reinfused. Several reinfusion systems are available. They significantly diminish net blood loss and blood transfusion requirements. Patients with good cardiac contractility who have the capacity to increase cardiac output readily will tolerate a hematocrit as low as 25%. Patients with severely restricted cardiac output should have their hematocrit maintained at 30%.

REOPERATION FOR BLEEDING

Reoperation for bleeding is necessary if:

1. Cardiac tamponade or compression has occurred due to undrained liquid blood or laminated clot.
2. Bleeding causes ongoing hypovolemia or anemia requiring excessive administration of blood. The latter must be qualified by the caveat that surgical exploration will not alleviate severe coagulopathy and should not be undertaken in its presence except for tamponade.

Classic cardiac tamponade is marked by high venous pressure, low arterial pulse pressure, and dramatic exacerbation of arterial hypotension with any further impairment to cardiac filling (e.g., increasing positive pressure inspiration or reverse Trendelenburg position). This classic syndrome warrants prompt reoperation, thorough removal of clotted as well as liquid blood, and exploration for a bleeding source. A less florid picture of restricted cardiac filling is encountered more often. Venous pressure may not be elevated because of hypovolemia. The hypovolemia is usually due to blood loss and is manifested as excessive chest drainage. If, at the time of chest closure, accumulated blood is not aspirated from the chest because of a desire to allow for defibrination and reinfusion, and if this volume is increased by antibiotic irrigation, there will be a large volume of chest drainage in the first 1 or 2 hours after operation. If tachycardia and hypotension accompany this high volume of early drainage, bleeding that warrants reexploration is likely. In the absence of tachycardia and hypotension (or in the absence of increasing need for vasopressors), significant bleeding is unlikely.

REFERENCES

1. Green GE: Use of internal thoracic artery for coronary artery grafting. *Circulation* 79:I-30–I-33, 1969.
2. Green GE, Swistel DG, Cameron AA: Bilateral internal thoracic artery surgery: 17 year experience. *Eur Heart J* 10:H57–H60, 1969.

CHAPTER 11
Pulmonary Complications

GEORGE E. GREEN

PATHOPHYSIOLOGY

Passage of blood through the oxygenator sets the stage for lung injury. Contact of blood with the polymer materials of the oxygenator activates proteolytic enzymes, complement, and leukocytes. Capillary permeability is increased,[1-3] and fluid leaves the vascular bed. The infusions required to maintain intravascular volume increases the total body fluid. The lungs share the burden. Pulmonary diffusion and compliance are diminished. Atelectasis, perfusion-ventilation mismatch, hypoxia, and increased pulmonary arterial resistance occur. In brief, lung function is impaired. Impairment can be minimized by minimizing fluid loading. If maximal cardiac output is pursued during the first few hours after heart-lung bypass, inordinate fluid loading will result. Much trouble can be avoided by judicious use of vasopressors to diminish the need for fluid. Limits of tolerance for vasopressors are indicated by skin color, temperature, and moisture; arterial pulse amplitude; urine output; and mixed venous oxygen saturation. As capillary permeability returns to normal, the need for vasopressors ceases. Fluid is mobilized from the extravascular space. Diuretics are required until pulmonary compliance (observed as inspiratory pressure of the respirator) is brought toward normal.

PHRENIC NERVE INJURY

Some reports of pulmonary morbidity following coronary bypass surgery implicate internal thoracic artery (ITA) grafts as an incremental risk factor.[4,5] The most extreme manifestation of pulmonary morbidity is the need for continuing mechanical ventilation. Such a need warrants evaluation of phrenic nerve function. Phrenic nerve palsy requires special, prolonged respiratory therapy. It is best recognized early. Orthopnea characterized by inward motion of the abdominal wall as the chest moves out is a sign of phrenic palsy. Diaphragmatic excursion in the 70° sitting position is normally 6 cm or more and can often be judged by physical examination. Motion that is severely diminished (less than 2 cm) or paradoxical (the diaphragm moves up with expansion of the chest wall) indicates phrenic nerve palsy. This should be documented by x-ray. Central or peripheral injury can be the cause. Differentiation can be made by transcutaneous phrenic nerve electrical stimulation. Whether peripheral or central, phrenic nerve palsy requires prolonged respiratory therapy based on extended use of a mechanical respirator or on the use of accessory muscles of respiration combined with postural control of diaphragmatic motion. The latter can be achieved during waking hours by maintenance of the upright position and during sleep by the use of a rocking bed (45° upright tilt, 15° downward tilt).[5]

Phrenic nerve palsy after coronary bypass surgery can have predisposing causes unrelated to the operation. Central (poliomyelitis, cerebral vascular ischemia) or peripheral factors (diabetes, osteoarthritis, herniated cervical disc, previous trauma) may play a role but are not controllable. Surgical technique is controllable and can minimize the incidence of phrenic nerve palsy, which has been recognized following cardiac surgery in 0.2 to 10% of cases.[6]

Cold injury to the phrenic nerve has been most extensively documented and has most commonly occurred after filling of the pericardium with saline slush or ice.[7] This can be readily avoided. Other surgical traumas—cutting, crushing, electrical, ischemic, traction—can be minimized. The phrenic nerve is juxtaposed to the proximal 2 cm of the ITA (Fig. 6–3). I deliberately separate it from the ITA. If the potential for injury to the phrenic nerve is not recognized, its vulnerability is increased. It is vulnerable during mobilization of the proximal 2 cm of the ITA and is especially vulnerable when the ITA is transected for use as a free graft. It is subject to injury when incisions are made in the pericardium for routing of ITA grafts and when traction sutures are placed in the posterior pericardium for exposure of the circumflex artery. Despite all these cautions, or perhaps because of them, phrenic nerve injury has not been a source of morbidity in any of the several thousand ITA grafts I have done over the past 22 years.

PLEURAL EFFUSION

Pleural effusions are relatively common. They are due in part to division of the lymphatics in the pleuropericardial folds. They tend to be a minor source of morbidity because they usually are not of sufficient volume to interfere with respiration. Effusions can be minimized by avoiding hypervolemia and by leaving chest tubes in place until drainage has diminished to less than 100 ml in an 8-hour period.

Chylous effusion is extremely rare. This is surprising in view of the fact that the origin of the ITA is close to the thoracic duct. Persistent chylous effusion warrants surgical exploration to identify and ligate the source of the chyle leak, evacuate loculated chyle, and decorticate and expand the lung.

REFERENCES

1. Smith EEJ, Naftel DC, Blackstone EH, et al: Microvascular permeability after cardiopulmonary bypass. *J Thorac Cardiovasc Surg* 94:225–233, 1987.
2. Haeffner-Cavaillon N, Roussellier N, Ponzio O, et al: Induction of interleukin-1 production in patients undergoing cardiopulmonary bypass. *J Thorac Cardiovasc Surg* 98:1100–1106, 1989.
3. Videm V, Fosse E, Mollnes ET, et al: Different oxygenators for cardiopulmonary bypass lead to varying degrees of complement activation in vitro. *J Thorac Cardiovasc Surg* 97:764–770, 1989.
4. Curtis J, Narvarawong W, Walls J, et al: Elevated hemidiaphragm following cardiac surgery: Incidence, prognosis and relationship to the use of topical ice slush. *Ann Thorac Surg* 48:764–768, 1989. Boca Raton, Fla, CRC Press, 1987.
5. Abd AG, Braun NT, Baskin MI, et al: Diaphragmatic dysfunction after open heart surgery: Treatment with a rocking bed. *Arch Intern Med* 111:881–886, 1989.
6. Fortune RL, Baron PJ, Fitzgerald JW: Atresia of the left main coronary artery: Repair with left internal mammary artery bypass. *J Thorac Cardiovasc Surg* 94:150–151, 1987.
7. Robiscek F, Duncan GD, Hawes AC, et al: Biological thresholds of cold-induced phrenic nerve injury. *J Thorac Cardiovasc Surg* 99:167–170, 1990.

CHAPTER 12

Wound Infection

GEORGE E. GREEN

INCREMENTAL RISKS

Internal thoracic artery (ITA) grafts have been described as an incremental risk factor for mediastinal or sternal infection in some surgical series but not in others.[1-4] Of those surgeons describing an increased risk, some report that the use of even one ITA is associated with increased infection.[5,6] Others report that the use of one ITA is not, but that the use of both ITAs is associated with an increased rate of infection.[7] Still others report that incremental risk appears only when both ITAs are used in subgroups of patients who are diabetic or obese or who need prolonged postoperative ventilatory support.[8,9]

In my practice, I have found no difference in infection rates between patients having exclusively saphenous vein grafts, one ITA graft, or two ITA grafts.[10] However, since 1985, comparison has not been possible because I have been routinely using both ITAs. Mediastinal or sternal infection has occurred in less than 2% of cases. The incidence of diabetes (insulin dependent = 18%) or marked obesity has not been different from that in series reporting higher infection rates.[11,12]

Why ITA use is a risk factor in some series but not in others has not been determined, but reasonable intuitive comments can be made. The "learning curve" was a term that haunted discussions of ITA surgery in the mid-1970s. At that time, it seemed to be a real deterrent to general use of the procedure. After 1983, when the dramatic preferential patency of ITA grafts was recognized, most surgeons negotiated the learning curve. However, in many surgical groups, the surgeon who mobilizes the ITA graft is always at the beginning of this curve—i.e., the newest, most junior staff member, who may seek to express surgical facility by speed. Rapid mobilization of the ITA is enhanced by cutting a wide, deep pedicle with a high-intensity current. The technique is simple and fast but leaves large areas of ischemic tissue. Some groups of patients are more resistant to infection than others. Nevertheless, I believe that surgical technique is sufficiently controllable to weigh significantly against the variability of patients' immune status. Surgical technique is the central issue when infection occurs after ITA mobilization.[13,14]

MANAGEMENT OF WOUND INFECTION

When infection occurs, early recognition and treatment is of prime importance. Unresolved infection near new vascular anastomoses can lead to dehiscence and exsanguination. Unresolved infection remote from new vascular anastomoses but in areas of vascularity can lead to disseminated sepsis. Unresolved infection in avascular areas leads to progressive necrosis.

Drainage of purulent fluid from a sternotomy incision within 10 days of operation is the most common presentation of major wound infection. It warrants complete surgical exploration (i.e., endotracheal anesthesia and removal of all sutures used for closure).

Drainage of serous or serosanguinous fluid should be scrutinized by Gram stain and culture. If these show the presence of bacteria, major wound infection is so likely that thorough exploration is warranted.

Drainage of serous or serosanguinous fluid containing no bacteria may be a harbinger of wound dehiscence, but also possibly of infection. Ongoing scrutiny of such wounds is indicated. If dehiscence becomes apparent, surgical exploration is warranted. If in the operating room no purulence is found and Gram stain shows no bacteria, the dehiscence should be repaired. If there is purulence or microscopic evidence of bacteria, the wound should be considered infected and treated as such.

The first of my patients who had wound infection after coronary bypass surgery had a small amount of purulent drainage from the middle of his sternotomy incision. Culture showed *Staphylococcus epidermidis*. A 2.5-mm sinus tract extended to the sternum. There was no wound tenderness. Low-grade fever existed. The patient was 200 miles from home and eager to go home. He was discharged from the hospital on the 10th postoperative day with a prescription for oral antibiotics and instructions for wound care. Six weeks after the operation, he was hospitalized at his local hospital because of high fever and severe chest discomfort. The sinus tract was still present and was draining small amounts of purulent material. Intravenous antibiotic therapy was begun. Bloody drainage occurred from the sinus tract and became increasingly profuse. Surgical exploration, undertaken to control the bleeding, terminated with exsanguination.

Many modalities for managing deep wound infection have been advocated. The one with the longest and best record is open drainage until the infection resolves. Leaving a sternotomy would open early after coronary bypass surgery mandates tracheal intubation and controlled positive-pressure ventilation. Positive end-expiratory pressure is of additional benefit. If respiration is not controlled, each inspiratory effort will separate the lungs further from the chest wall and mediastinum, compounding the problem of wound healing.

Exploration of wound infection early after coronary bypass surgery begins with general anesthesia and tracheal intubation. All cutaneous, subcutaneous, fascial, and sternal sutures are removed. Purulence is aspirated and necrotic tissue is resected. Posterior drainage tubes are placed in each pleural space. A small catheter for delivery of antibiotic irrigation is placed in the anterior mediastinum. (Sufficient positive pressure should be applied to the lungs to appose them to the chest wall and mediastinum.) Dressings are held in place with a loosely applied elastic chest binder. Neuromuscular blockade is not reversed. The patient is transferred to the intensive care unit with controlled ventilation. Morphine is administered every 2 to 4 hours to keep the patient deeply obtunded and to facilitate controlled ventilation with positive end-expiratory pressure. Appropriate antibiotics are administered by intravenous and mediastinal routes. Fever, leukocytosis, and purulence usually resolve rapidly. Clean granulation tissue usually becomes apparent quickly and covers all surfaces within 7 days.

Closure of the wound is then appropriate. If controlled positive-pressure ventilation has been maintained, and if exploration and debridement were undertaken early, there will be no "dead space" as the wound is closed. The sternum is closed with wires. A single layer of simple interrupted monofilament retention sutures is used to approximate loosely the soft tissues of the upper abdominal wall and the chest wall. The dermis may be further approximated with additional simple interrupted sutures. The pleural drains and mediastinal infusion catheter are left in place. Positive-pressure ventilation is continued for 24 hours, and the patient is then weaned from the respirator. Mediastinal antibiotic infusion is continued for 48 hours. Infusion and drainage tubes are then removed. Intravenous antibiotic therapy is continued until the patient leaves the hospital—usually 1 week after wound closure.

Muscle and Omental Flaps

If effective positive-pressure ventilation has not been maintained, or if there has been substantial loss of sternum, cartilage, or soft tissue, space will exist that must be obliterated by well-vascularized tissue. If the space is small, the simplest procedure is closure with pectoral myocutaneous flaps.[15] Larger spaces will not be filled by myocutaneous flaps and are best filled with a pedicled graft of omentum based on the right gastroepiploic artery.[16] Such grafts easily extend to the neck. Space between the costal arch and the diaphragm must not be overlooked. Persistent space behind the costal arch can result in very troublesome chondritis. The space is easily filled by omentum.

If omentum is not available, inferior (caudal) spaces can be filled with reverse rectus muscle flaps. Anastomoses of the lower intercostal arteries with the superior epigastric artery usually afford good vascularity to the rectus muscle despite prior mobilization of the ITAs.[17] Superior (cephalad) spaces that are too large to be closed by advancement of pectoral myocutaneous flaps can be filled by rotation of pectoral muscle flaps based on the thoracoacromial arteries.[17]

Open drainage, tracheal intubation, and positive-pressure ventilation seem an awesome departure early in the postoperative course. But I am convinced that this is the safest and most expeditious way to manage this grave complication. Its gravity and the virtue of open drainage are emphasized by a review of 6,505 consecutive patients who had coronary bypass surgery at the Cleveland Clinic between 1985 and 1987. Seventy-two patients (1.1%) developed deep wound infection. Hospital mortality for this group was 14%. During the year following hospital discharge, they experienced an additional 14% mortality. Three modes of surgical management were used: debridement followed by open chest and late sternal closure (12 patients), debridement and closure over irrigation and drainage catheters (41 patients), and debridement and primary closure with muscle or omental flaps (19 patients). Mortality was 17% and 16% for the latter two groups, respectively. There was no mortality in the group treated by debridement, open chest, and late sternal closure. There was no significant difference in the length of the hospital stay for the three modes of treatment, perhaps because 10 of the 60 patients treated by methods other than debridement, open chest, and late closure required reoperation for sternal instability and persistent sepsis. Another review of 3,229 consecutive adult open heart surgery patients focused on the optimal initial treatment for sternal wound infections.[18] It concluded that "if open treatment is used as the initial treatment for all patients with a deep wound infection, definitive therapy would begin earlier, with near zero mortality rate and a cure rate approaching 100%."[19]

Not all infections are manifested within 10 days of operation. Infections discovered later are also best treated by prompt removal of all suture material, thorough exploration, and debridement. If the lungs are adherent to the chest wall and mediastinum, mechanical ventilation is not required. Open treatment is continued until the entire wound is covered with granulation tissue. Surgical closure or spontaneous closure ensues.

REFERENCES

1. Galbut DL, Tradd EA, Dorman MJ, et al: Seventeen-year experience with bilateral internal mammary artery grafts. *Ann Thorac Surg* 49:195–201, 1990.
2. Engelman RM, Williams CD, Gouge TH, et al: Mediastinitis following open-heart surgery: Review of two years' experience. *Arch Surg* 107:772–778, 1973.
3. Tector AJ, Davis L, Gabriel R, et al: Experience with internal mammary artery grafts in 298 patients. *Ann Thorac Surg* 22:515–519, 1976.
4. Nkongho A, Luber JM, Bell-Thomson J, et al: Sternotomy infection after harvesting of the internal mammary artery. *J Thorac Cardiovasc Surg* 88:788–789, 1984.
5. Culliford AT, Cunningham JN, Zeff RH, et al: Sternal and costochondral infections following open heart surgery: A review of 2594 cases. *J Thorac Cardiovasc Surg* 72:714–726, 1976.
6. Gross EA, Esposito R, Harris LJ, et al: Sternal wound infections and use of internal mammary grafts. *Proc NY Soc Thor Surg* 2:3, 1990.
7. Hazelrigg SR, Wellons HA, Schneider JA: Wound complications after median sternotomy: Relationship to internal mammary artery grafting. *J Thorac Cardiovasc Surg* 98:1096–1099, 1989.
8. Loop FD, Lytle BW, Cosgrove DM, et al: Sternal wound complications after isolated coronary artery bypass grafting: Early and late mortality, morbidity, and cost of care. *Ann Thorac Surg* 49:179–187, 1990.

9. Kouchoukos NT, Wareing TH, Murphy SF, et al: Risks of bilateral internal mammary artery bypass grafting. *Ann Thorac Surg* 49:210–219, 1990.

10. Cameron A, Kemp H, Green GE: Bypass surgery with the internal mammary artery graft: 15 year follow up. *Circulation* 74(Suppl III):31–36, 1986.

11. Green GE, Sosa JA, Cameron A: Prospective study of feasibility of routine use of multiple internal mammary artery anastomoses. *J Cardiovasc Surg* 30:643–647, 1989.

12. Green GE, Swistel DG, Cameron AA: Bilateral internal thoracic artery surgery. *Eur Heart J* H57–H60, 1989.

13. Nishida H, Grooters RK, Merkley DF, et al: Postoperative mediastinitis: A comparison of two electrocautery techniques on presternal soft tissues. *J Thorac Cardiovasc Surg* 99:969–976, 1990.

14. Mills NH: Discussion of risks of bilateral IMA grafting. *Ann Thorac Surg* 49:218, 1990.

15. Jeevanandam V, Smith CR, Rose EA, et al: Single-stage management of sternal wound infections. *J Thorac Cardiovasc Surg* 99:256–263, 1990.

16. Lovich SF, Iverson LI, Young JN, et al: Omental pedicle grafting in the treatment of postcardiotomy sternotomy infection. *Arch Surg* 124:1192–1194, 1989.

17. Nahai F, Rand RP, Hester TR, et al: Primary treatment of the infected sternotomy wound with muscle flaps: A review of 211 consecutive cases. *Plast Reconstruct Surg* 84:434–441, 1989.

18. Fortune RL, Baron PJ, Fitzgerald JW: Atresia of the left main coronary artery: Repair with left internal mammary artery bypass. *J Thorac Cardiovasc Surg* 94:150–151, 1987.

19. Prevosti LG, Subramainian VA, Rothaus KA: A comparison of the open and closed methods in the initial treatment of sternal wound infections. *J Cardiovasc Surg* 30:757–763, 1989.

CHAPTER **13**

ITA Graft Spasm, Inadequacy, and Malfunction

GEORGE E. GREEN

SPASM

Mention of spontaneous internal thoracic artery (ITA) graft "spasm" as a cause of myocardial injury after ITA-coronary bypass surgery is so frequent that it is surprising to find only three published reports—one surgical and two medical. Scrutiny of these reports leads to doubt that they do in fact document spontaneous ITA graft spasm as a cause of myocardial injury.

The surgical paper, written by Sarabu et al.,[1] reported two patients. The first had elective single-vessel bypass surgery because of symptomatic restenosis at the site of a previous transluminal angioplasty. The report stated: "Nine hours postoperation, the patient precipitously experienced ventricular fibrillation and hemodynamic collapse refractory to external electrical defibrillation. . . . The chest was reopened and inspection revealed profound spasm of the distal 2 cm of the IMA graft immediately above its anastomosis. [The] patient was replaced on cardiopulmonary bypass, after which defibrillation was accomplished successfully. Minimal contraction of the anterolateral wall was observed. . . . Postmortem examination revealed massive recent myocardial infarction of the septum and the anterolateral wall in the distribution of the LAD artery." It seems unlikely that the massive infarction described post mortem was due to acute postoperative loss of perfusion from the ITA graft. It is well established that 12–18 hours are required for histological changes of infarction (edema, neutrophil invasion) to be evident. The cause of the spasm at the site of the ITA anastomosis is open to question. The authors contend that the spasm was unrelated to surgical trauma. They describe the ITA at the site of anastomosis as being initially 3 mm in diameter. This diameter is unusually large. Trauma can disrupt the vessel wall and increase its size. Initially, there may be very good flow. Later behavior may not be so good. Endothelial injury profoundly alters endothelium-dependent vasomotor tone.[2] The fact that papaverine, an endothelium-independent vasodilator, mitigated the spasm does not preclude trauma as the initiating event.

When preparing ITA grafts for anastomosis, I have seen separation of the intima from the media that I did not appreciate until I looked at the graft with 8× magnification. Separation of intima from media can occur during dissection of the ITA from the chest wall. It can also be caused by transection of the ITA with an inappropriate scissor, by dilatation, or by clamping of the distal end of the ITA. If areas of separation are not excised back to normal coherent artery, trouble may ensue.

The second patient in the report of Sarabu et al. was a 65-year-old man with progressive angina. The report stated: "Saphenous vein grafts were placed to the diagonal branch of the LAD, the marginal branch of the circumflex, and the right posterior descending arteries. A three millimeter left IMA was anastomosed to the distal LAD artery. The patient came off bypass without difficulty, demonstrating cardiac output of six liters. After chest closure and as the patient was being transferred to the intensive care unit, he experienced acute hemodynamic compromise." Ventricular fibrillation occurred. "The chest was reopened, and internal defibrillation was performed successfully. Left ventricular contractility was observed to be diffusely poor and severe spasm of the distal one centimeter of the IMA graft was found. A papaverine soaked sponge was immediately placed over the IMA graft and increasing infusions of dopamine, epinephrine, and nitroglycerin were begun. After fifteen minutes, the IMA graft was restored to its original size and the patient stabilized completely." It seems highly unlikely that spontaneous postoperative spasm of the ITA graft was responsible for the global cardiac injury described. The cause of the spasm is not explained. The fact that it was relieved by topical papaverine does not exclude surgical trauma as a possible cause. This paper, the sole surgical report claiming to document spontaneous idiopathic postoperative spasm of the ITA as a cause of myocardial injury, seems flimsy ground for the contention.

It is distressing to hear surgeons and cardiologists frequently attribute postoperative hemodynamic instability and ST-segment elevation to idiopathic ITA spasm. A favorable response to calcium channel blockers is taken as proof of ITA spasm. Sarabu and co-authors conclude their paper by recommending long-term calcium channel blockade to alleviate "spasm" of the ITA when ST-segment elevation is observed. Calcium channel blockade is helpful in relieving myocardial ischemia. A more reasonable concept of relief of adverse changes by calcium blockade is relief of myocardial ischemia, not necessarily relief of graft spasm. More likely causes of myocardial ischemia after ITA anastomosis are arterial trauma, suture stricture, torsion, or tension. Surgeons would do better to scrutinize their technique than to advocate indefinite calcium blockade. Spasm, if observed, is more likely to be due to surgical graft injury than to bad luck.

The cardiological literature describing spontaneous spasm of ITA grafts consists of two reports. "Angiographic Demonstration of Spasm in a Left Internal Mammary Artery Used as a Bypass to the Left Anterior Descending Coronary Artery" was published in 1988.[3] I am grateful to Dr. Bernard L. Segal for letting me study the original angiograms. The paper cites the case of a patient undergoing angiography for angina that recurred 1 year after saphenous vein graft to the right coronary artery and left internal thoracic artery anastomosis to the left anterior descending coronary artery. Angiograms revealed a patent saphenous vein graft to the right coronary artery but stenosis in this artery beyond the vein graft. The initial injection of the left ITA (LITA) showed a normal LITA. Subsequent injection showed a smooth, tapering stenosis in the proximal third of the graft remote from the catheter tip, interpreted as spasm of the graft. Review of the original angiogram compels me to interpret it differently. I think it shows the following:

1. Dissection of the subclavian artery with persistent dye in the wall of the subclavian artery (Fig. 13–1A).
2. Extension of the dissection from the subclavian artery down to the proximal third of the ITA (Fig. 13–1B–D).

The angiographic study terminated with a demonstration of the "spasm." Resolution of the spasm was postulated as the reason for lack of persistent signs and symptoms of ischemia. If, as I believe, traumatic dissection was the cause of the deformity, reentry of dissection into the true lumen is the likely explanation for resolution of the ischemia. I have observed such a sequence during angiographic study of a patient I operated on.

"Spontaneous Reversible Spasm in an Internal Mammary Artery Graft Causing Acute Myocardial Infarction" was published in 1989.[4] Dr. Jeffrey Hartzler, the co-author, helped me obtain the angiograms for review. The case reported is of a 60-year-old man who had LITA anastomosis to the left anterior descending artery and saphenous vein grafting to the lateral circumflex and right coronary arteries. Nine years after operation, with no premonitory symptoms, he experienced an anterior myocardial infarction (Q waves V1–V4). Angiography was performed 7 days after the infarction. At that time, the patient was taking no cardiac medications. Occlusion of the left anterior descending artery distal to the first septal branch was demonstrated. Opacification of the ITA graft showed that "a discrete aneurysm was present in the proximal third of the artery. Shortly thereafter the artery tapered to a long tubular zone that was approximately ninety percent stenotic in several areas. The distal left internal mammary artery and distal left anterior descending artery appeared normal." After discharge, exertional angina prompted referral to Dr. Hartzler for angioplasty of the ITA graft. "As per routine, the patient was premedicated with 5 mg of isosorbide dinitrate sublingually and 5 mg of verapamil intravenously." Selective visualization of the LITA showed no narrowing in the graft. The proximal aneurysm in it was unchanged, as was the left anterior descending artery. The authors conclude that "complete resolution of the long tubular narrowing in the body of the left internal mammary artery strongly suggests reversible spasm as the cause of the anterior myocardial infarction." I believe the initial angiogram shows intramural dissection that spirals to a long narrowing (Fig. 13–2A–D). The final angiogram appears to be compatible with reentry of dissection into the true lumen of the ITA.

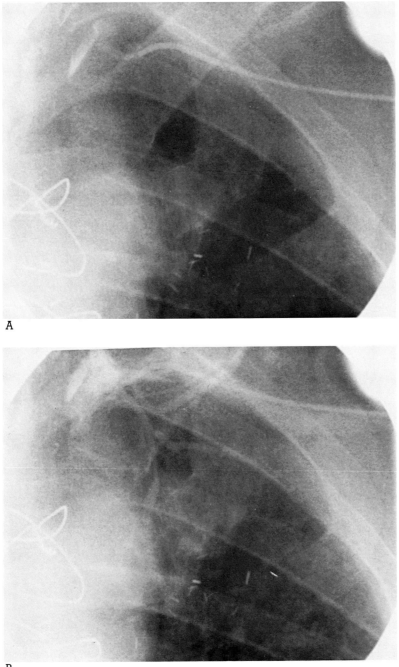

A

B

FIGURE 13-1 A: Pocketing of dye indicates dissection of the subclavian artery. **B–D:** Dissection extends into the proximal third of the ITA, simulating or causing spasm.

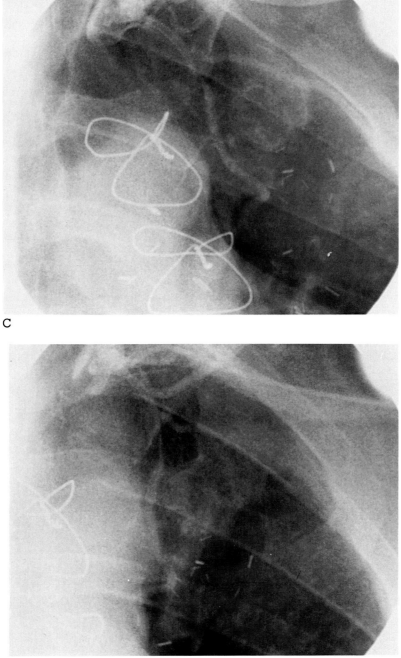

C

D

FIGURE 13–1 Continued

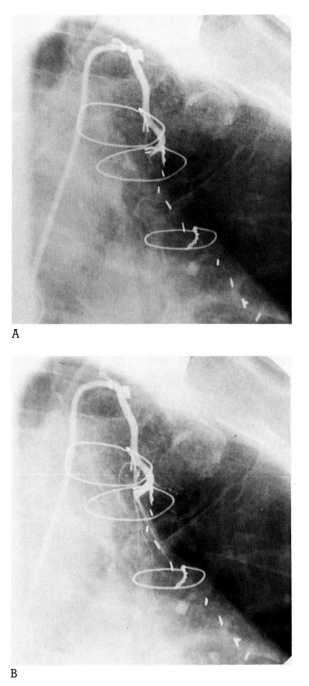

A

B

FIGURE 13–2 A–D: Narrowing in this ITA graft may be due to dissection rather than spasm.

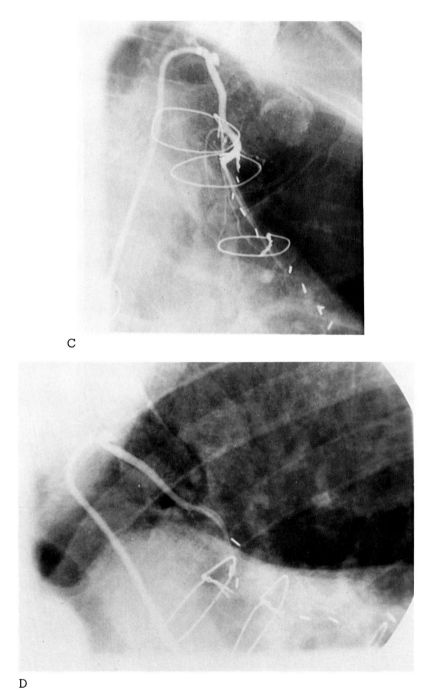

C

D

FIGURE 13–2 Continued

The presence of the saccular aneurysm of the proximal ITA makes the case particularly complex. Aneurysms of small blood vessels are conspicuous causes of thromboembolism. The myocardial infarction that preceded the first restudy is more likely to have been due to microembolism than to spontaneous ITA spasm.

These four cases, which comprise all the available evidence for the contention that spontaneous idiopathic spasm of ITA grafts has caused myocardial ischemia do not prove their contention.

ITA ADEQUACY AND MALFUNCTION

Reports of inadequacy or malfunction of ITA grafts emphasize that the remarkable capacity of these grafts to increase progressively in size and flow does not warrant magical thinking.

Ellis Jones' "Catastrophic Consequences of Internal Mammary Artery Hypoperfusion"[5] illustrates that even an ITA significantly smaller than the coronary artery to which it is anastomosed will not immediately increase in size to provide unrestricted flow. Similarly, when an ITA is used for sequential anastomoses, its size should equal the sum of the sizes of the coronary arteries to which it is anastomosed. I am compelled to add to Jones' observations that flow from ITA grafts should be scrutinized prior to anastomosis to eliminate the use of damaged grafts—regardless of whether they are free or pedicled. Finally, when anastomosing arteries 1.5 mm in diameter, I believe it is unrealistic not to use high magnification (8×).

Reports such as "Kinking of Internal Mammary Grafts"[6] by Brenot et al. emphasize that the geometry of the graft cannot be ignored simply because the graft is an ITA and resistant to thrombosis.

It is also important to know that, on rare occasions, obstruction to the subclavian inflow of a pedicled ITA graft can develop after operation; can cause impairment of flow into the coronary system; and can cause progressive ischemia by reversal of flow—coronary to subclavian steal. Such conditions not only can arise, they can be documented by arteriography and corrected surgically.[7]

REFERENCES

1. Sarabu MR, McClung JA, Fass A, et al: Early postoperative spasm in left internal mammary artery bypass grafts. *Ann Thorac Surg* 44:199–200, 1987.
2. Chesbro JH, Fuster V, Webster MWI: Endothelial injury and coronary vasomotion. *J Am Coll Cardiol* 14:1191–1192, 1989.
3. Kong B, Kopelman H, Segal BL: Angiographic demonstration of spasm in a left internal mammary artery used as a bypass to the left anterior descending coronary artery. *Am J Cardiol* 61:1363, 1988.
4. Stone GW, Hartzler GO: Spontaneous reversible spasm in an internal mammary artery graft causing acute myocardial infarction. *Am J Cardiol* 64:822–823, 1989.

5. Jones EL, Lattouf DM, Weintraub WS: Catastrophic consequences of internal mammary artery hypoperfusion. *J Thorac Cardiovasc Surg* 98:902–907, 1989.

6. Brenot P, Mousseaux E, Relland J: Kinking of internal mammary grafts: Report of two cases and surgical correction. *Cathet Cardiovasc Diagn* 14:172–179, 1988.

7. Granke K, Van Meter CH, White CJ, et al: Myocardial ischemia caused by postoperative malfunction of a patient internal mammary coronary arterial graft. *J Vasc Surg* 11:659–604, 1990.

CHAPTER 14

Arterial Grafts Other than the ITA in Coronary Bypass Surgery

Frequent late failure of saphenous vein grafts has prompted attempts to achieve complete revascularization with arterial grafts. In these attempts, other arteries in addition to internal thoracic arteries (ITAs) usually need to be used. They are used in the hope that they may share the favorable fate of the ITAs.

Historical perspective may not promote new developments, but it can be helpful in evaluating them. In the early 1970s, a few surgeons preferred total revascularization with arterial grafts. Their preference was based primarily on the desire to avoid the early failures of saphenous vein grafts due to thrombosis or progressive subintimal fibrosis.[1] Secondary reasons for preferring arterial revascularization were theoretical. They fell into one of three groups. One was based on the idea that pedicled grafts are more viable than free grafts. The second was based on the idea that ITA grafts were relatively immune to early thrombosis or fibrotic stricture because their closer size match to the coronary arteries avoided the turbulent flow seen in large saphenous vein grafts. The third was the idea that arteries might be better than veins just because they were arteries.

The first arterial graft other than the ITA to be advocated for coronary bypass surgery was the splenic artery pedicled graft.[2] The technical difficulty of dissecting the artery from the pancreas and spleen, and the potential morbidity of pancreatitis or splenectomy, prevented widespread use of this graft. I did use the procedure. My reasons for abandoning it were three. First, I was troubled by the atherosclerotic changes seen in the artery as it was being separated from the pancreas. Second, although bringing the pedicled graft through the diaphragm posed no technical problem, I was concerned about potential distortion by postoperative postural changes or abdominal distention. Finally, angiographic evaluation of a procedure I thought technically perfect showed closure of the graft—not a meaningful statistic, but for me a meaningful deterrent.

Radial artery grafts were introduced by Carpentier et al. in 1973.[3] They advocated these grafts because they were arterial grafts and comparable in size to the coronary arteries. They were easier to mobilize and suture than the ITA. They were free grafts and, as such, had more versatility than the pedicled ITA. Soon after its introduction, postoperative angiography showed stricture in the body of the graft. Carpentier et al. stated that stricture could be prevented by thorough mechanical dilatation of the prominent muscular wall. This did not help, and radial artery grafts were abandoned because angiographic restudy showed severe fibrotic stricture or occlusion in most cases.[4]

The right gastroepiploic artery, mobilized from the greater curvature of the stomach, was first used for myocardial revascularization by Bailey.[5] He advocated it as a pedicled implant into the posterior myocardium. Its use ceased when direct arterial anastomosis replaced the indirect technique. It was reintroduced to myocardial revascularization in 1984 by Pym. He used it as a pedicled bypass graft to arteries of the posterior surface of the heart when leg veins were unavailable or when extensive disease of the ascending aorta made aortic clamping seem unsafe.[6] In advocating the use of this vessel, Pym referred to a study by Larsen et al. of atherosclerosis of gastric arteries.[7] Pym's report implies that the study by Larsen et al. showed that "the right gastroepiploic artery . . . is usually freer of atherosclerosis than other vessels such as the splenic artery." Larsen et al.'s excellent study of gastric atherosclerosis in 103 cadavers did not include sections from any part of the right gastroepiploic artery. The closest their study came to this artery was the gastroduodenal artery behind the pylorus. That area was chosen because the study focused on factors contributing to gastroduodenal hemorrhage. Degrees of atherosclerotic plaque were recorded that would impair the ability of arteries to contract if penetrated by ulcer. Such degrees of atheromatous plaque were recorded in 7 of 103 gastroduodenal arteries. Although the study was not concerned with potential flow reserve, the histology of the arteries was described. In addition to 7 arteries that showed major atheromatous plaques, 58 showed thickening of the intima; the degree of thickening was not specified.

Summa et al. were the next to report on the use of the right gastroepiploic artery in coronary bypass surgery.[8] Their "basic study" included histology and angiography. The histological survey consisted of several sections of the right gastroepiploic arteries of five patients who had undergone gastrectomy. The authors reported: "None of the specimens displayed the histological characteristics of arteriosclerosis." The angiographic aspect of their basic study consisted of reviewing 100 celiac angiograms randomly selected from the files of the department of general surgery. The length and diameter of the gastroepiploic arteries were recorded, and "only one celiac angiogram demonstrated stenosis of the gastroepiploic artery." It is not stated that each study included at least two projections. It is probable that each study included only one. Such technique is inadequate for evaluating atherosclerosis of the coronary arteries and for evaluating arteries to be used as coronary bypass grafts.

Lytle et al. reported the Cleveland Clinic experience with 32 patients who had gastroepiploic grafts between 1985 and 1988.[9] Nine of these patients had angiography 1 to 13 months after the operation. These nine grafts were patent. Lytle et al.'s report included histological examination of distal segments of the right gastroepiploic artery from 18 patients. "None of the segments exhibited atherosclerosis and they were histologically indistinguishable from segments of the IMAs." It is impossible to derive confidence from that statement. The ITA is an elastic artery. Its media is composed predominantly of multiple elastic lamina. Smooth muscle cells, elastin, and collagen are interspersed. The gastroepiploic artery is a muscular artery. Its media is composed predominantly of smooth muscle cells. Elastin and collagen are interspersed. It is hard to imagine that the gastroepiploic artery segments studied by Lytle et al. were "histologically indistinguishable from segments of the IMAs." Their report goes on to state: "Our data and the studies by others have shown that the IMA and the gastroepiploic artery are histologically similar and that atherosclerosis intrinsic to either vessel is uncommon." The study to which Lytle et al. refer is that of Larsen et al. Contrary to the contentions of Pym and Lytle et al., that work does not mention the right gastroepiploic artery at all.

Casual study of the gross and microscopic appearance of the right gastroepiploic artery in autopsy specimens causes me to view its use in coronary bypass surgery with reserve. Gross atherosclerosis of the right gastroepiploic artery in autopsy specimens is not uncommon. It can easily be overlooked during surgical mobilization of a fatty pedicle that contains the artery. Moreover, microscopic examination of this muscular artery shows its internal elastic lamina to be frequently disrupted. Its intima is usually thickened (Fig. 14–1A,B).

Use of the right gastroepiploic artery in the absence of a suitable ITA or saphenous vein is reasonable. Prospective evaluation of it is desirable. But until significant numbers of late studies are available, preferential use of the right gastroepiploic artery is based on wishful thinking. One drawback in using the right gastroepiploic artery is that its use precludes later use of the greater omentum as a pedicled graft, if needed.

The inferior epigastric artery was first used in coronary bypass surgery by Puig in 1987. In 1990 he reported the use of the graft in 22 patients.[10] Seventeen of the patients were restudied angiographically early after operation. Fifteen of the 17 grafts were patent. The inferior epigastric artery is histologically similar to the right gastroepiploic artery. Its media is predominantly composed of smooth muscle cells and collagen. Its wall is somewhat thinner than that of the right gastroepiploic artery.[11] It is mobilized through an infraumbilical midline incision. The anterior rectus sheath is incised lateral to the midline. The rectus muscle is retracted. The artery is dissected from the anterior surface of the posterior rectus sheath. At the level of the umbilicus, it breaks into multiple branches. These anastomose with ramifications of the superior epigastric branch of the ITA. As the dissection is taken toward the origin of the inferior epigastric artery, the posterior rectus sheath disappears and the artery lies on preperitoneal fat. It can be transected at its origin from the external iliac artery or with a wedge of the anterior wall of the external iliac artery. The latter procedure is facilitated by a short incision parallel and

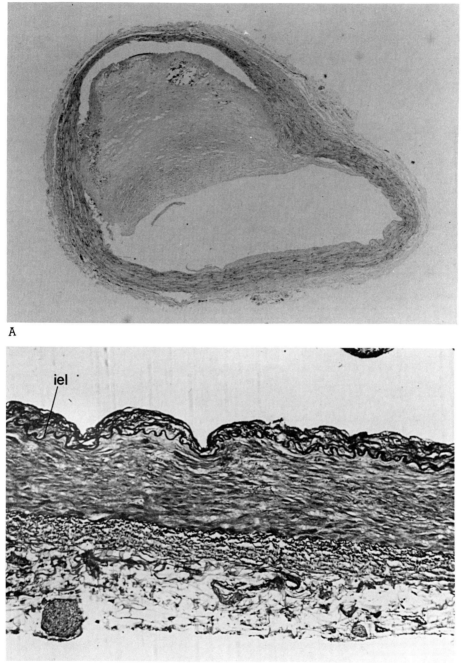

A

B

FIGURE 14–1 A: Marked atheromatous change in a right gastroepiploic artery. **B:** Fragmentation of the internal elastic lamina (IEL) of the right gastroepiploic artery and intimal thickening.

cephalad to the inguinal ligament. Such dissection provides a graft of about 15 cm. Both internal epigastric arteries can be used. To date there have been no reports of abdominal wall ischemia from the use of the internal epigastric artery, even when used in combination with the ipsilateral ITA. Collateral arterial flow is from lower intercostal and lumbar branches of the aorta.

Although to date there are only two reports other than Puig's on the use of the inferior epigastric artery,[11,12] its use is spreading rapidly. More will be heard about it.

REFERENCES

1. Dilley RJ, Hons BS, McGeachie JK: A review of the histologic changes in vein to artery grafts with particular reference to intimal hyperplasia. *Arch Surg* 123:691–696, 1988.
2. Edwards WS, Lewis CE, Blakely WR: Coronary artery bypass with internal mammary and splenic artery grafts. *Ann Thorac Surg* 15:35–40, 1973.
3. Carpentier A, Guermonprez JL, Deloche A: The aorta to coronary radial artery graft: A technique for avoiding pathological changes in grafts. *Ann Thorac Surg* 16:111–121, 1973.
4. Curtis JJ, Stoney WS, Alfred WC Jr: Intimal hyperplasia: A cause of radial artery to aorto-coronary bypass graft failure. *Ann Thorac Surg* 20:628–635, 1975.
5. Bailey CP, Hirose T, Brancato R: Revascularization of the posterior (diaphragmatic) portion of the heart. *Ann Thorac Surg* 2:791–805, 1966.
6. Pym J, Brown PM, Charette EJ: Gastroepiploic-coronary anastomosis. *J Thorac Cardiovasc Surg* 94:256–259, 1987.
7. Larsen E, Johansen A, Anderson D: Gastric arteriosclerosis in elderly people. *Scand J Gastroenterol* 4:387–389, 1969.
8. Summa H, Fukumoto H, Atsuro T: Coronary artery bypass grafting by utilizing in situ right gastroepiploic artery: Basis study and clinical application. *Ann Thorac Surg* 44:394–397, 1987.
9. Lytle BW, Cosgrove DM, Ratliffe NM: Coronary artery bypass grafting with the right gastroepiploic artery. *J Thorac Cardiovasc Surg* 97:826–831, 1989.
10. Puig LZ, Ciongolli W, Cividanes GVL: Inferior epigastric artery as a free graft for myocardial revascularization. *J Thorac Cardiovasc Surg* 99:251–255, 1990.
11. Van Som AM, Smedts F, Vincent JG: Comparative anatomic studies of various arterial conduits for myocardial revascularization. *J Thorac Cardiovasc Surg* 99:703–707, 1990.
12. Vincent JG, Van Som AM, Skotmicki SH: Inferior epigastric artery as a conduit in myocardial revascularization: The alternative free arterial graft. *Ann Thorac Surg* 49:323–325, 1990.

Epilogue

Revascularization of the heart using the internal thoracic arteries (ITAs) is now accepted as the most effective technique for surgical revascularization. This technique has helped to focus attention on the artery. There is increasingly widespread appreciation of Sims' discovery of the unique histology of the ITA. Sims showed that the internal elastic lamina (IEL) of the ITA is different from that of the coronary artery, and that fragmentation of the IEL of the coronary artery leads to atherosclerosis. I believe that integrity of the IEL will increasingly be considered the hallmark of arterial integrity. Further study may show how the iel of ITAs is maintained and how those of coronary arteries can be enhanced.

It will be a pleasing paradox if surgical treatment of coronary artery disease helps lead to a mode of prevention.

Index